Diagnostic Parasitology

for

Veterinary Technicians

Edited by

Joann Colville, DVM
Department of Veterinary Science/Microbiology
North Dakota State University
of Agriculture and Applied Science
Fargo, North Dakota 58105

Book Editor: Paul W. Pratt, VMD
Production Manager and Cover Design:
Elisabeth S. Stein

American Veterinary Publications, Inc.
5782 Thornwood Drive
Goleta, California 93117

© 1991

Library of Congress Card Number: 90-085892
ISBN 0-939674-32-7

Printed in the United States of America

Authors

Lowell J. Ackerman, DVM
Mesa Veterinary Hospital
858 N. Country Club Drive
Mesa, AZ 85201

Thomas R. Bello, DVM, PhD
Sandhill Equine Center
635 Niagara Road
Southern Pines, NC 28387

Larry A. Capitini, BVSc, MRCVS
Clinical Instructor
Department of Veterinary
    Preventative Medicine
Ohio State University
Columbus, OH 43201

Alan M. Fudge, DVM
California Avian Laboratory
6114 Greenback Lane
Citrus Heights, CA 95621

Sayed M. Gaafar, DVM, MS, PhD
Professor Emeritus –
Department of Parasitology
Purdue University
2620 Newman Road
West Lafayette, IN 47906

Peter J. Ihrke, VMD
Professor
Department of Medicine
Chief – Dermatology Service
Veterinary Medical Teaching Hospital
School of Veterinary Medicine
University of California
Davis, CA 95616

Lynn P. Schmeitzel, DVM
Associate Professor
Department of Urban Practice
College of Veterinary Medicine
University of Tennessee
Knoxville, TN 37901

Dawn A. Shaffer
Supervisor
Department of Veterinary Pathology
College of Veterinary Medicine
University of Missouri
Columbia, MO 65211

Charles A. St. Jean, BSc, DVM
Professor
Department of Veterinary Technology
Columbus State Community College
Columbus, OH 43215

William F. Wade, DVM, MS, PhD
Territory Veterinary Clinic
7315 US Hwy 20
Galena, IL 61036

Joseph E. Wagner, DVM
Professor and Chairman
Department of Veterinary Pathology
College of Veterinary Medicine
University of Missouri
Columbia, MO 65211

Contents

1

Introduction

W.F. Wade and S.M. Gaafar

A complete review of parasitology (the study of parasites) is beyond the scope of this book. Only the general types of parasites and their products that may be found by diagnostic procedures will be described.

The reference sources listed at the end of the various chapters can provide more information on parasitology and specific parasites.

Parasites and Parasitism

Parasites are organisms that live on (external parasites) or within (internal parasites) an animal, deriving their nutrition and protection at the expense of the animal. The infected animal is called the host.

Parasites have many different life cycles. Life cycle refers to how an organism develops and reproduces itself. Each parasite has a distinctive life cycle comprised of various developmental stages, which can be in the same or in different hosts. The life cycle of successful parasites has at least one stage at which it can pass from one host to the next (be transmitted), and this is frequently the stage detected by diagnostic procedures. This transmitted stage may leave its host through excretions, such as feces or urine, or it may be transmitted to its next host by an insect, such as mosquitoes transmitting heartworms in dogs.

Protozoa

Protozoa are one-celled organisms, some of which are parasitic in domestic animals. There are many different groups of protozoa living in many different host tissues, but the technician in a veterinary practice will most likely find protozoa either in blood samples (hemoprotozoa) or fecal samples (intestinal protozoa). Their life cycles vary from simple to very complex. In the complex life cycles, there are a few stage names that are important to understand.

Trophozoite refers to a stage of the life cycle of an intestinal protozoan parasite that is capable of feeding and movement. Some intestinal protozoans form a stage called a *cyst*, which is incapable of movement. Usually in the intestinal protozoa that form cysts, trophozoites are the forms that live within the animal, while the cysts are passed out in the feces. The cysts are acquired by another host, which then becomes infected. Examples of this type of intestinal protozoa include *Balantidium coli* and *Giardia canis*. The *oocyst* is the rigid-walled cyst stage of a special group of intestinal protozoa called coccidia, examples of which are *Eimeria* and *Isospora*.

Most hemoprotozoa seen in the United States are diagnosed in RBC in blood smears. The RBC containing the hemoprotozoa are acquired by blood-sucking arthropods (*eg*, ticks) and transmitted to another animal. An example of this group is *Babesia*. Trypanosomes are another group of hemoprotozoa, occasionally found in the United States, that live in the blood but outside of RBC. They are 3-10 times as long as a RBC is wide and boat-like in shape, with a thin, whip-like flagellum used for swimming. They are also transmitted by blood-sucking arthropods.

Trematodes

Trematodes (flukes) are flatworms with unsegmented leaf-like bodies. In domestic animals in the United States, most adult fluke parasites are found in the intestines, liver or lungs. In these locations the flukes lay microscopic eggs that are passed out in the feces. These eggs may be seen using fecal examination tests described in the next chapter. Many fluke eggs have a small part of the shell that is separated from the rest by a rim, this small part being called the operculum or lid. Eggs of a few other types of parasites have this structure, but it is most common among flukes. The eggs contain a larva or "young fluke," which hatches and develops in intermediate hosts, such as snails and fish. Later, another host acquires the larva (frequently by consuming the intermediate host as a contaminant of its food or water), and the fluke matures and begins producing eggs in the new host. Examples of flukes include the lung fluke of dogs and cats (*Paragonimus kellicotti*) and liver flukes of cattle and sheep (*Fasciola hepatica, Fascioloides magna, Dicrocoelium dendriticum*).

Cestodes

The cestodes (tapeworms) are also flatworms but, unlike the flukes, they are ribbon-like and divided into a long chain of proglottids (segments) strung out like train cars behind a scolex ("head"), by which it is attached to the host's intestinal wall. Many tapeworms release proglottids one at a time (or in short chains) into the feces; these proglottids may be seen with the naked eye. Several types of tapeworms have proglottids, which are light in color and can move on their own, that clients sometimes describe as white "worms" crawling in the feces or on the hair of their animals.

The proglottids of many tapeworms contain eggs when they are passed in the feces. The eggs contain larvae called hexacanth embryos, "hexa-" meaning 6 and "-canth" meaning hooks; therefore, within the egg, 6 hooks may be seen, aiding identification. The eggs are eaten by an intermediate host, in which the larva develops. The type of intermediate host depends on the type of tapeworm; they may be arthropods, fish or mammals. Larvae that live in mammals develop into "bladder worms," which are like fluid-filled balloons in the tissues of the intermediate host. If the intermediate host is eaten by a new host, a new adult tapeworm develops in that host's intestine. Examples of tapeworms include the fringe tapeworm of cattle (*Thysanosoma actinioides*) and the flea tapeworm of dogs and cats (*Dipylidium caninum*).

Nematodes

The nematodes (roundworms) are a very important group of parasites, different types of which may be found in almost any tissue of the body. In domestic animals the main types are roundworms in the intestines, lungs, kidneys, urinary bladder and blood. The life cycles are very diverse and complicated; however, usually either the eggs or larvae of roundworms in the intestines and lungs are found in the feces and the eggs of roundworms in the kidney and bladder are found in the urine. Examples of intestinal roundworms include large roundworms (ascarids), hookworms (*Ancylostoma, Uncinaria stenocephala*) and whipworms (*Trichuris*). Urinary roundworms include swine kidney worms (*Stephanurus dentatus*), and respiratory roundworms include the lungworms of cattle and sheep (*Dictyocaulus, Muellerius capillaris*).

Roundworms of the blood are a special group, of which the canine heartworm (*Dirofilaria immitis*) is an important example. The adult females of this group lay a small, worm-like microfilaria. The microfilaria can be seen in the blood with a microscope and is usually about 40 times the diameter of a RBC in length. Microfilariae of canine heartworms are taken up with the blood by a blood-sucking mosquito, in which they develop to larvae that are transmitted to other dogs by the bite of the mosquito.

Acanthocephalans

The acanthocephalans (thorny-headed worms) are relatively less common intestinal parasites with complicated life cycles. Their eggs are sometimes seen during fecal examinations of pigs or dogs. Adults may occasionally be seen in the intestine at necropsy.

Arthropods

The arthropods are a very large group of organisms that represent over 75% of all the living creatures in the world. Fortunately, only a few are parasitic. Examples of those include blood-sucking flies, mites, ticks and fleas. Most arthropod parasites of domestic animals are discussed in the chapters on external parasites; however, some insect larvae live as internal parasites of domestic animals, such as the stomach bot of horses. As we have noted, blood-sucking arthropods (*eg,* mosquitoes, ticks) are very important in transmission of some internal parasites.

2

Common Laboratory Procedures for Diagnosing Parasitism

W.F. Wade and S.M. Gaafar

The term "parasites" represents many different types of organisms that live in and on animals, feeding on tissues or body fluids or competing directly for the animal's food. These parasites have an amazing variety in their size and appearance. Whereas none of the bacteria or viruses are visible to the naked eye, parasites include organisms that range in size from those too small to be seen without a microscope, up to organisms measuring more than a foot long. Parasites show great variety in the places in which they live in animals and the ways in which they are transmitted from one animal to another. Due to these wide variations in size and life cycles, there is no one particular diagnostic test to identify all parasites.

This chapter discusses procedures a veterinary technician may be asked to perform as an aid to diagnosis of internal and external parasitisms. Generally these procedures are used to detect the presence of parasites or their products, such as their eggs or larvae, on the skin or in the animal's excretions or blood. Some of these procedures are not in common use in most veterinary practices but are mentioned because they may be useful to technicians employed in diagnostic or research laboratories.

It is important to note that these tests are not totally reliable. Sometimes an animal may be infected with parasites but because infection is slight, no detectable stages are being shed or the wrong test is used, no parasites are detected. For this reason, practitioners use not only these tests but also the animal's history, clinical signs and other laboratory tests, such as blood values, to arrive at a specific diagnosis of internal parasitism.

DIAGNOSIS OF PARASITISM OF THE DIGESTIVE TRACT

W.F. Wade and S.M. Gaafar

The following procedures can be used as aids in diagnosis of parasitism of the throat, stomach, liver, pancreas and intestines. They can also be used for diagnosis of parasitic infections in other parts of the body, when the eggs or larvae are passed out by way of the digestive tract (*eg*, lung parasites).

Collection of the Fecal Sample

Veterinary technicians usually do not have the opportunity to collect fecal samples and must rely on samples brought in by clients or samples the practitioner may collect during farm calls. Regardless of how they are obtained, it is important to have fresh feces with which to work. Practitioners realize this, but it may need to be emphasized to clients. The need for fresh feces stems from rapid development and changes that occur in some common parasite eggs once they are passed from the animal, as well as the death of some protozoa that can be recognized by their movement. If fresh feces cannot be obtained, advise the client to refrigerate the sample (no more than 24 hours).

Small Animal Samples

For small animal fecal samples, it is better to ask that the client actually witness the animal defecating to ensure the source of the sample and to note any straining, blood in the feces or other problems. Immediately upon receipt of the sample, the container should be properly labeled with the owner's name, the animal's name, and the time and date of collection. In laboratories that process a large number of fecal samples, it is sometimes convenient to assign each sample a number to ensure that samples are processed in the order in which they are received and to aid in record keeping.

It is best to provide clients with disposable containers in which to place the feces. Waxed-paper ice cream cups, with a 3- to 5-oz capacity and sealing lids, work well for this. The minimum amount of feces for examination is 2 g (about 1/2 tsp); however, about a half a Dixie cup full allows the technician to more easily observe for any blood, mucus or large parasites.

Large Animal Samples

Large animal fecal samples should, if possible, be collected directly from the animal's rectum. While wearing a disposable plastic glove, the practitioner making rectal examination of horses or cattle can grasp a handful of feces and then turn the glove inside out while removing it. The open end is then tied with a knot and the glove is labeled with the owner's name, the animal's name or number, the date and time of collection.

Samples from pigs, feedlot cattle or other grouped animals are often pooled samples, *ie,* several samples are taken from a pen, without the specific animal of origin being known. These samples should be as fresh as possible and each sample should represent only one group of animals in direct contact with one another. Disposable plastic bags make good containers for pooled large animal fecal samples. These samples should be labeled with the owner's name, the specific location of the pen, the number of animals, and the date and time of collection. It is always important to have clean containers that can be tightly sealed to prevent loss of samples.

Any fecal sample that cannot be examined within an hour after its collection should be refrigerated to slow or stop the parasite's development and reduce unpleasant odors.

Examination of the Fecal Sample

Several procedures commonly used to examine feces for parasites are described in this section. Before attempting to apply these procedures, a few points should be considered:

- *Always handle fecal samples carefully.* Some parasites, bacteria and viruses in animal feces are a threat to human health. When examining the samples, the technician should always wear appropriate clothing and rubber or plastic gloves, if available. If these are not available, hands should be washed thoroughly with a disinfectant soap after performing the tests. Under no circumstances should food or drink be consumed in the area where these tests are performed.

- *Always clean up immediately after the tests have been performed.* Leaving spilled material or dirty glassware lying about creates a source of contamination and could lead to serious human or animal infections.

- *Always keep good records.* A notebook should be kept in the laboratory area and every sample should be listed by the date, owner's name and the animal's name or number. Any observations about the appearance of the fecal sample, as well as any parasites found, should be written down immediately. Finding no parasites should be recorded; otherwise it will be thought the test has not yet been done. In recording negative findings, write "NPS" (No Parasites Seen). Always transfer results from the notebook to the animal's permanent record.

Gross Examination of Feces

Several characteristics of feces should be recorded and relayed to the attending practitioner.

Consistency: Are the fresh feces soft, watery (diarrhea) or very hard (constipation)? This judgment varies with the animal's species. For instance, cattle feces are normally softer than those of horses or sheep.

Color: Always record unusual fecal colors. For instance, light-gray feces may indicate excessive fat in the feces, a sign of poor intestinal absorption.

Blood: In fresh feces, blood may appear dark brown to black and tar-like, or the red color that is associated with fresh blood. Blood may indicate severe parasitism, as well as other intestinal disease. Its presence is very important to record, as it assists the practitioner in identifying certain diseases.

Mucus: Mucus on the surface of the feces may be associated with parasitism or other disease and should be noted.

Age of the Feces: If the feces appear old and dry, this should be recorded. In old samples, parasites may be distorted or unrecognizable.

Parasites: Some parasites or parts of parasites are large enough to see with the naked eye. Probably the most common are the proglottids of tapeworms, but there may also be larval arthropods or entire adult worms.

Tapeworm segments (proglottids) in fresh feces are shown in Figure 1. These should be gently picked from the feces with forceps and examined. Segments of 2 common tapeworm segments found in the feces of dogs and cats are shown in Figure 2. Their shape, size and movement, if any, aid identification. Figure 3 illustrates tapeworm segments from ruminants and horses. Segments from ruminants are often seen in short chains in fresh feces. Swine in the United States do not have tapeworm segments in their feces.

Occasionally clients bring in dried-out tapeworm segments they have found in their animal's bedding or hair. To identify these segments from their shape, they must be rehydrated by soaking for 1-4 hours in a Petri dish or small saucer containing water or physiologic saline.

The technician should always attempt to identify the genus of the segments so the practitioner can use this information in control and treatment of the tapeworm infection. The structure of the segment can help differentiate tapeworms. For example, with *Dipylidium caninum*, the tapeworm of dogs and cats that is transmitted by fleas, you can observe, with magnification, a "pore" (opening) on either side of the segment. Segments of tapeworms of the genus *Taenia*, which use mammals (rodents and rabbits) as intermediate hosts, have a single pore on each segment. Tapeworm segments are definitively identified by identifying the eggs they contain.

Segments of some uncommon tapeworm species do not contain eggs, and some of the common types of segments may have already expelled their eggs. If there is doubt whether the mate-

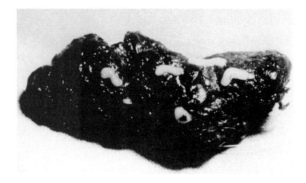

Figure 1. Fresh dog feces containing tapeworm segments.

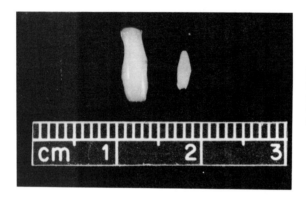

Figure 2. Mature segments of the most common tapeworms of dogs and cats, *Taenia* (left) and *Dipylidium* (right).

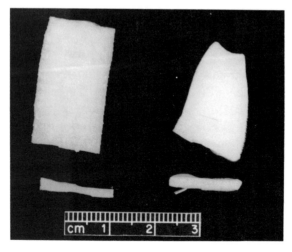

Figure 3. Chains and individual, mature segments of tapeworms of cattle, *Moniezia* (left), and horses, *Anoplocephala* (right).

Examination of Tapeworm Segments for Eggs

Materials: thumb forceps
dissection needles (hypodermic needles work well)
microscope slides and coverslips

1) Remove the segment from the feces with thumb forceps and place in a drop of water on the slide.

2) Using the dissection needles, pull the segment into several small pieces on the slide. Crush and mix the pieces with the drop of water.

3) Remove the pieces of segment with the forceps and place the coverslip over the water on the slide.

4) Examine the slide with a microscope (as described in the next section). Compare the appearance of any eggs found with photographs of common tapeworm eggs.

---

rial is really a tapeworm segment, the material may be crushed between 2 microscope slides and examined with a microscope to see if the tissue has small mineral deposits (calcareous bodies), which are found only in tapeworm material (Fig 4).

Other types of parasites are large enough to be seen in animal feces. These include adult worms forced out of their host by drug treatments or overcrowding by their fellow parasites (Fig 5). Horse feces may contain "bots," which are the larvae of a certain type of fly. Bots normally live in the stomach of horses and are passed in the feces to complete their life cycle outside the body (Fig 6).

Figure 4. Microscopic calcium deposits (calcareous bodies) in tapeworm tissue. (140X)

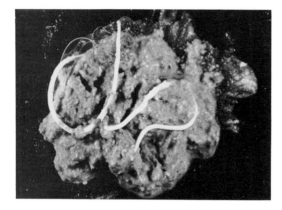

Figure 5. Two roundworms (*Toxocara canis*) in canine feces after treatment.

Figure 6. Larvae (bots) of bot flies in equine feces.

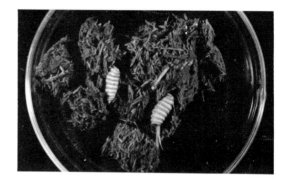

Feces may also contain nonparasitic fly larvae called maggots (Fig 7). These maggots do not live within the animal but instead develop from eggs laid by adult flies after the feces have been passed. Maggots are seen in feces voided more than 12 hours previously and should not be mistaken for internal parasites.

In general, when the technician cannot identify parasite-like material found in the feces, the material should be sent to a diagnostic laboratory for identification. Specimens should be preserved in 70% alcohol or 10% formalin and shipped as described later in this chapter.

Microscopic Examination of Feces

Microscopes vary widely in features and magnifications they can provide. For parasitologic work, objective lenses with magnification power of 4X, 10X and 40X are useful. Oil-immersion

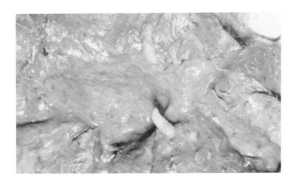

Figure 7. Free-living fly larvae (maggots) in 2-day-old
bovine feces.

objectives (*eg*, 100X) are occasionally used in veterinary practice. A mechanical stage is preferable and convenient for parasitologic work because it allows for smooth movement and a
thorough search of the slide. Regardless of how the slide is
moved, the area under the coverslip must be thoroughly
searched.

To search the slide thoroughly, begin using an objective that
magnifies at least 10X (with experience you may be able to scan
the slides more rapidly at 4X). The edge of the coverslip can be
used for adjusting the coarse focus and fecal debris under the
coverslip used for fine focus adjustment. Each circular area of
the slide seen through the microscope is called a field. The slide
should be moved so the field follows the pattern of arrows shown
in Figure 8. Each time the edge of the coverslip is reached, a
piece of debris at the edge of the field (in the direction of the

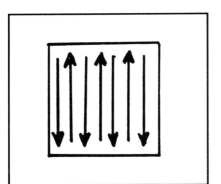

Figure 8. Scheme of movement of the
microscopic field to thoroughly examine
the area under the coverslip.

search) should be identified. The slide is then moved until the piece of debris is at the opposite edge of the field. In this fashion, every field scanned slightly overlaps the previous and every area under the coverslip is examined. While the slide is being scanned in this manner, it is important to continually move the fine focus knob back and forth slightly to aid visualization of parasite eggs or cysts not in a single plane of focus. When a parasite egg is seen at low magnification, higher-power objectives may be used to more closely examine it.

Calibrating the Microscope

The size of the various stages of many parasites is often important for correct identification. Some examples are *Trichuris* versus *Capillaria* eggs and *Dipetalonema* versus *Dirofilaria* microfilariae. Accurate measurements are easily obtained by using a calibrated eyepiece on the microscope. Calibration must be performed on every microscope to be used. Each objective (lens) of the microscope must be individually calibrated.

Instruments: The stage micrometer is a microscope slide etched with a 2-mm line marked in 0.01-mm (10-μ) divisions (Fig 9). Note that 1 micron (μ) equals 0.001 mm.

The eyepiece scale is a glass disc that fits into and remains in one of the microscope eyepieces. This disc is etched with 30 hash marks spaced at equal intervals (Fig 9). The number of hash

Figure 9. Stage micrometer and eyepiece scale used to calibrate a microscope.

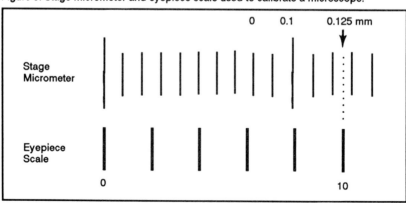

marks on the disc may vary with different manufacturers, but the calibration procedure does not change.

The stage micrometer is used to determine the distance in microns between the hash marks on the eyepiece scale for each objective lens of the microscope being calibrated. This information is recorded and labelled on the microscope for future reference.

Procedure: Start on the low power (10X) and focus on the 2-mm line of the stage micrometer. Note that 2 mm equals 2000 μ. Rotate the eyepiece so that the hash-mark scale is horizontal and parallel to the stage micrometer scale (Fig 9). Align the "0" point on both scales.

Determine the point on the stage micrometer aligned with the "10" hash mark on the eyepiece scale. In Figure 9, this point is at 0.125 mm on the stage micrometer.

Multiply this number by 100. In our example, 0.125 x 100 = 12.5 μ. This means that at this power (10X), the distance between each hash mark on the eyepiece scale is 12.5 μ.

Repeat these steps at each magnification (10X, 40X, 100X). Record the information on a label and attach it to the calibrated microscope. For example,

Objective	Distance Between Hash Marks (μ)
10X	12.5
40X	2.5
100X	1.0

Direct Smear

The simplest method of microscopic fecal examination for parasites is the direct smear, which consists of a small amount of feces placed directly on a microscope slide. The advantages of this procedure are the short time and minimal equipment needed, as well as the small amount of fecal sample required. Some practitioners make direct smears with only the amount of feces that clings to a rectal thermometer after taking the animal's temperature. The direct smear allows the technician to see

---

Direct Smear Procedure

Materials: microscope slide and coverslip
applicator stick or toothpick
(optional: Lugol's iodine, diluted 1:5 with distilled water)

1) Place a drop of water or physiologic saline in the middle of a slide and an equal amount of feces next to it. A drop of iodine may also be used to help highlight protozoa (see Examination of Feces for Protozoa).

2) Thoroughly mix the feces and water or saline (and iodine) with the applicator stick to form a homogenous emulsion.

3) Make a smear on the surface of the slide. Be sure the smear is not too thick. The print on a piece of newspaper placed under the slide should be visible through the smear.

4) Remove any large fecal particles with the stick and place a coverslip over the smear. The coverslip should sit evenly over the smear.

5) Examine the smear with the microscope for parasite eggs or larvae.

---

eggs and larvae undistorted by the procedures discussed later. The main disadvantage of this procedure is its inaccuracy. Such a small piece of feces may not contain the parasite larvae or eggs the animal is harboring and the animal may be incorrectly assumed to be free of parasites. This procedure also leaves a lot of fecal debris on the slide, which may confuse the technician.

Concentration Methods for Fecal Examination

As mentioned above, the greatest disadvantage to the direct smear procedure is the small amount of feces used, which greatly reduces the chance of finding parasite material. To overcome this problem, methods have been developed to concentrate parasitic material from a larger fecal sample into a small volume, where it may be examined microscopically. There are 2 primary types of concentration methods used in veterinary practices: flotation and sedimentation.

Fecal Flotation

Flotation methods are based on differences in specific gravity of parasite eggs, cysts and larvae and that of fecal debris. Specific gravity refers to the the weight of an object (*eg*, the parasite egg) as compared to the weight of an equal volume of pure water.

Most parasite eggs have a specific gravity between 1.100 and 1.200 (g/ml), while tap water is only slightly higher than 1.000. Therefore, parasite eggs are too heavy to float in tap water. To make the eggs float, a liquid with a higher specific gravity than that of the eggs must be used. Such liquids are called flotation solutions and consist of concentrated sugar or various salts added to water to increase its specific gravity. Flotation solutions usually have specific gravities between 1.200 and 1.250. In this range, fecal material, which has a specific gravity of 1.300 or greater, does not float. The result of using flotation solutions is that parasite eggs float to the surface of the liquid and large particles of fecal material sink to the bottom.

Sugar, salt and sodium nitrate solutions are the most commonly used in veterinary practices. Sugar solution is less efficient (floats fewer eggs) than sodium nitrate solution and is

---

Preparation of Flotation Solutions

Sugar flotation solution (Sheather's solution)

Determine the amount of sugar solution required and use about half that amount of water. Use a pot (such as a cooking pot) that can hold the amount of solution you want. Heat the water but be careful not to let it boil. Add granulated pure cane sugar (table sugar) to the water while stirring. About 454 g (1 lb) are needed for every 355 ml (12 oz) of water. Add 6 ml of formalin per 454 g of sugar or 1 g of crystalline phenol for every 100 ml of solution; these chemicals serve as preservatives. The solution's specific gravity should always be checked with a hydrometer (Fig 10), an instrument available from scientific supply houses (*eg*, Scientific Products, 1210 Waukegan Rd, McGaw Park, IL 60085). If the specific gravity is below the desired range (1.200-1.250), add more sugar until the hydrometer reads in this range. If the specific gravity is above 1.250, add water until the proper reading is obtained.

Sodium nitrate solution

Add about 315 g of sodium nitrate for every liter of water, while stirring. Heating is not necessary but hastens the dissolution process. Adjust the solution to a specific gravity of 1.200-1.250 as discussed for the sugar solution.

Zinc sulfate solution

Add about 386 g of zinc sulfate to 1 L of water, while stirring. Heated water speeds dissolution of the zinc sulfate. Adjust to a specific gravity of 1.200-1.250 with a hydrometer.

Saturated sodium chloride solution

Add table salt to boiling water until the salt no longer dissolves, and settles to the bottom of the pot. There is no need to adjust the specific gravity, as it cannot go above 1.200 with this solution.

messy to work with, but it is readily available and cheap, does not distort roundworm eggs, and floats an adequate percentage of the eggs. Sodium nitrate solution is the most efficient but it forms crystals and distorts the eggs after a time. Sodium nitrate is sometimes difficult to acquire but can be purchased through chemical supply houses. Sodium nitrate solution is used in commercial fecal diagnostic kits (see below) and may be purchased already prepared in the form of refill bottles for these kits. Whatever the source, sodium nitrate solution is more expensive than sugar solution.

Saturated sodium chloride solution is the least desirable flotation solution. It corrodes laboratory equipment, forms crys-

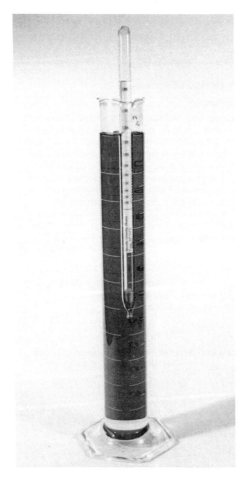

Figure 10. Measuring the specific gravity of a flotation solution with a hydrometer.

Simple Flotation Procedure

Materials: flotation solution
    shell vial (straight-sided vials 1.25-2.0 cm in diameter and
    5.0-7.5 cm tall)
    waxed paper cups (90-150 ml) or 100-ml beakers
    cheesecloth or gauze squares (10 x 10 cm) or metal-screen
    tea strainers
    wooden tongue depressors or applicator sticks
    microscope slides and coverslips

1) Take about 2 g (1/2 tsp) of the fecal sample and place it in the cup. Add about 30 ml of flotation solution, using a tongue depressor, and make an emulsion by thoroughly mixing the solution with the feces until no large pieces of feces remain.

2) Bend the side of the cup into a spout and cover that spout with the cheesecloth. Pour the emulsion through the cheesecloth into the vial. If using the tea strainer, pour the contents of the cup through the strainer and into a second cup, then pour the contents of the second cup into the vial.

3) Fill the vial to the top and slightly overfill it, so that a dome of liquid (a meniscus) rises above the lip of the vial without overflowing down the side (Fig 11). If there is not enough fluid in the cup to fill the vial, a small amount of fresh flotation solution may be added.

4) Place a coverslip gently on top of the fluid and allow it to settle on the liquid dome.

5) Allow the coverslip to remain undisturbed on top of the vial for 10-20 minutes (sugar solution requires longer than sodium nitrate). If removed before this time, all of the eggs may not have time to float to the top. If left for more than an hour, some eggs may become waterlogged and begin to sink or become distorted.

6) Remove the coverslip carefully, picking it straight up, and immediately place it on the microscope slide. When placing it on the side, be sure to hold the coverslip with one edge tilted slightly up and allow it to settle level on the slide gradually; this avoids air bubbles under the coverslip.

7) Examine the area of the slide under the coverslip with a microscope, as previously described, and record any eggs, larvae or whole parasites seen.

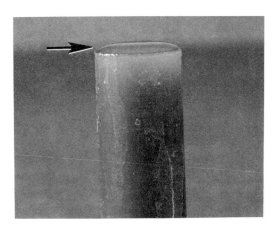

Figure 11. A shell vial filled with flotation solution, show-ing the meniscus (arrow).

tals on the slide and distorts the eggs severely. Because it only reaches a specific gravity of 1.200, some heavier eggs may not float. However, it is inexpensive, easily made and readily available. Zinc sulfate solution is similar in efficiency to sugar solution but is relatively more difficult to obtain.

Simple Flotation: The simple flotation method is probably the second most common parasitologic test performed in veterinary practices, after the direct smear. The object of the test is to float the parasite eggs to the top of the tube of flotation solution, which is covered by a microscope coverslip. The eggs adhere to the coverslip, which is removed from the liquid and examined with a microscope. This method is less efficient than the centrifugal flotation described below but does not require a centrifuge.

Some companies have packaged a simple flotation kit consisting of prepared flotation solution, disposable plastic vials and strainers. Two examples are Ovassay (Pitman-Moore) and Fecalyzer (Evsco) (Fig 12). Both of these use sodium nitrate flotation solution. Instructions for their use are included with these kits. The main disadvantage of these kits is their expense.

Centrifugal Flotation: The centrifugal flotation procedure more efficiently recovers parasite eggs and cysts, and requires less time than the simple flotation procedure. However, it requires a centrifuge capable of holding 15-ml tubes and produc-

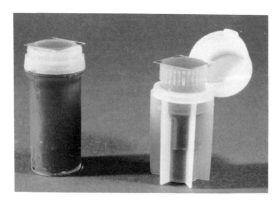

Figure 12. Two commercial fecal flotation kits. Ovassay (left) and Fecalyzer (right).

Centrifugal Flotation Procedure

Materials: (same as for simple flotation, but excluding shell vials)
    15-ml centrifuge tubes
    wire loop (as used for bacteriology) or glass rounded-end rod

1) Prepare the fecal emulsion as described for simple flotation.

2) Strain the emulsion through the cheesecloth into the centrifuge tube and fill the tube nearly to the top. If the centrifuge holds the tubes at a fixed angle, the tube should not be filled so high that the liquid runs out when placed in the centrifuge. Always balance the centrifuge by placing a tube of equal weight, containing another sample or water, in the opposite tube holder. Be sure all tubes are marked so they can be identified after centrifugation.

3) Centrifuge the tubes for 5 minutes at 400-650 gravities. For many centrifuges, this is about 1500 revolutions per minute (rpm).

4) Remove the tube from the centrifuge and gently place it in a test tube rack. A wire loop (bent at a 90-degree angle to the handle) or a glass rod is then touched to the surface of the liquid. The drop of fluid contained in the loop or on the end of the rod is then transferred to the microscope slide (Fig 13). Apply a coverslip and examine microscopically as previously described.

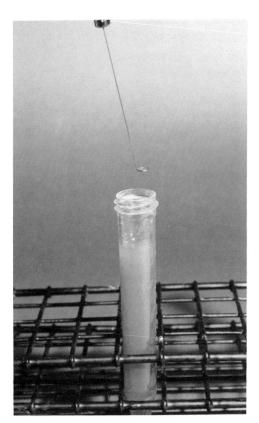

Figure 13. Use of the bacteriologic loop to transfer a drop from the top of the fecal flotation emulsion after centrifugation. Note that the loop is bent at a 90-degree angle to the handle.

ing centrifugal force of 400-650 gravities (most tabletop centrifuges produce this force).

Fecal Sedimentation

Sedimentation procedures concentrate both feces and eggs at the bottom of the liquid, which is usually water. Sedimentation detects most parasitic eggs but is not as good as flotation for providing a clear sample for microscopic examination. Sedimentation is mainly used to detect eggs or cysts that have too high a specific gravity to float or that would be severely distorted by flotation solution.

Sedimentation can be used for roundworm and tapeworm eggs, but there is usually too much fecal debris hiding the eggs to make it worthwhile. For that reason, this procedure is not used routinely and has its greatest use in suspected fluke infections. Fluke eggs are somewhat denser and sometimes larger than roundworm eggs. Some fluke eggs float in flotation solutions, while others do not. Some laboratories increase the specific gravity of their flotation solutions to 1.300 to ensure recov-

---

Sedimentation Procedure

Materials: waxed paper cups (90-150 ml) or beakers (100 ml)
cheesecloth or gauze squares (10 x 10 cm) or tea strainers
wooden tongue depressors
centrifuge and 15-ml centrifuge tubes
Pasteur pipettes and pipette bulbs
microscope slides and coverslips
(optional: Lugol's iodine diluted 1:5 in water)

1) Using a tongue depressor, mix about 2 g of feces with tap water in a cup or beaker. Strain the mixture through the cheesecloth or strainer into a centrifuge tube as described for centrifugal flotation.

2) Balance the centrifuge tubes and centrifuge the sample at about 400 gravities (about 1500 rpm). If a centrifuge is unavailable, allow the mixture to sit undisturbed for 20-30 minutes.

3) Pour off the liquid in the top of the tube without disturbing the sediment at the bottom.

4) Using the pipette and bulb, transfer a small amount of the top layer of sediment to a microscope slide. If the drop is too thick, dilute it with a drop of water. Lugol's iodine solution may be used for dilution instead of water, to aid in identification of protozoan cysts. Apply a coverslip to the drop. Repeat the procedure using a drop from the bottom layer of the sediment.

5) Examine both slides microscopically as described previously.

ery of fluke eggs by the flotation technique. The problem with use of flotation methods for recovery of fluke eggs is that the eggs may be damaged by the high concentration of the solution and become hard to identify.

Quantitative Fecal Examination

All of the procedures described previously have been qualitative, which means they only reveal whether parasites are present or not. Quantitative procedures indicate the number of eggs or cysts present in each gram of feces. These procedures are an indication of how many adult parasites are present within the host (the severity of the infection). The procedures are not completely accurate because different species of parasites produce different numbers of eggs. Also, the most severe signs of disease often are produced by young parasites that have not yet started to produce eggs or larvae.

Several procedures are used to estimate numbers of parasite eggs or cysts per gram of feces, including the Stoll egg count technique, the modified Wisconsin flotation method and the McMaster technique. Few veterinary practices perform quantitative tests, but they are often used in research laboratories. Of these tests, the McMaster technique is the most accurate and most commonly used, and is described below.

Examination of Feces for Protozoa

All of the previous procedures for microscopic fecal examination are useful for detection of cysts of intestinal protozoa. However, some protozoa do not form cysts and pass in the feces as trophozoites. Cyst-forming protozoa may also pass trophozoites in the feces in large numbers when the host has diarrhea. Trophozoites lack the rigid wall of cysts, and collapse and become difficult to recognize in flotation solutions.

To observe live trophozoites, a fecal smear should be prepared as previously described, but physiologic saline must be used to dilute the feces. Trophozoites are recognized by their movement, which varies among different groups of protozoa. *Balantidium coli*, a parasite of people, pigs and dogs, moves in a slow, tumbling fashion. *Giardia*, which is found in several species of animals, swims with a jerky motion. Trichomonads, also found in several different hosts, appear to wobble and have a sail-like structure that ripples as they move. Amoebae, found in people and dogs, move by extending part of their cell body (a pseudopod) and moving the rest of the body after it.

Many methods have been used to stain and/or preserve intestinal protozoa. The simplest method to stain cysts is a direct smear stained with an iodine solution (as described under the direct smear procedure). This method does not preserve the sample but highlights any protozoa in the smear, making their identification easier. Several different iodine solutions are avail-

---

McMaster Technique

Materials: McMaster counting chamber slide (Pet-Check Laboratories, Prairie Village, KS)
waxed paper cups or beakers
graduated cylinder
set of scales, weighing in grams
sugar flotation solution
wooden tongue depressors
test tubes, greater than 3-ml capacity
1-ml pipettes

1) Using the scales, weigh exactly 2 g of the fecal sample into a cup. With the graduated cylinder, measure exactly 28 ml of water and pour into the cup. Mix the feces and water together thoroughly, making sure no large pieces remain. If the feces are hard, allow them to soak for a few minutes before mixing.

2) Use the pipette to place exactly 1 ml of sugar solution into the test tube. Then use the same pipette to add 1 ml of the fecal mixture to the test tube. Thoroughly mix the solutions together by pipetting them in and out of the pipette or by shaking the tube. Do not use the same pipette for different fecal samples.

3) Use the pipette to take the mixture out of the test tube and completely fill the 2 chambers of the counting slide (Fig 14).

4) Allow the counting chamber slide to sit undisturbed for 20 minutes, which allows the eggs and cysts to float to the top of the solution in the chamber.

5) Over each chamber is an etched square divided into 6 equal columns. Place the slide on a microscope stage and focus on the etched lines with the scanning objective. The 10X objective may be used to count eggs or cysts but the thickness of the slide and chamber makes use of higher-power objectives impractical. Count all the eggs or cysts seen within the etched square, keeping a separate count for each different species of egg or cyst seen.

6) The area marked off by the square over each chamber represents a specific volume of solution (0.15 ml) in the chamber. The dilutions have been worked out so that to determine the number of eggs (or cysts) of each species per gram of feces, the number counted in both chambers is multiplied by 100 (multiply by 200 if only one chamber was counted). Record the species and the number, followed by EPG (eggs per gram).

Figure 14. A McMaster counting chamber slide being filled with fecal emulsion.

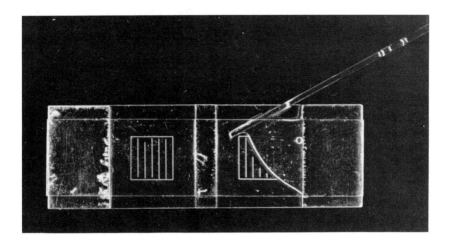

able for staining. Lugol's iodine is sometimes used in veterinary therapeutics and may already be on hand in a practice.

Fecal smears containing protozoal trophozoites may be allowed to dry and then stained with Giemsa, Wright's or Diff-Quik stain (Scientific Products). Once stained in this manner, the slides may be sent to a diagnostic laboratory for identification of the organism.

There are many other procedures for the concentration, staining and preservation of intestinal protozoa, including merthiolate-iodine-formaldehyde (MIF) solution, polyvinyl alcohol, iron hematoxylin and others. These procedures are generally too complex and time consuming for use in veterinary practice.

Preparation of Lugol's Iodine Solution

Before preparing this solution, the technician should remove all jewelry, as the solution can permanently stain precious metals.

Dissolve 10 g of potassium iodide in 100 ml of distilled water in a glass beaker. Then add 5 g of powdered iodine crystals to the solution and stir until all of the iodine has dissolved. This is therapeutic-strength (5%) Lugol's; it should be stored in an amber bottle, away from light. To use for staining, this solution must be diluted by adding 1 part of the 5% Lugol's solution to 5 parts of distilled water. The solution must be remade every 3 weeks because it deteriorates.

Fecal Culture

Fecal culture is used in diagnostic parasitology to differentiate parasites whose eggs and cysts cannot be distinguished by
examination of a fresh fecal sample. As an example, the eggs of
large strongyles in horses are very similar to those of small
strongyles. To distinguish between them, feces containing
strongyle eggs are allowed to incubate at room temperature for
several days while the larvae hatch from the eggs. The newly
hatched larvae can then be identified.

Roundworm Eggs

The procedure for culture of roundworm eggs in feces is
simple; however, identifying the larvae once they are recovered
is much more tedious. Technicians required to culture and
identify roundworm larvae are referred to the procedure below.

Coccidial Oocysts

Another type of fecal culture that has some use in veterinary
practices is sporulation of coccidial oocysts. Sporulation is a
process of development that takes place within the oocyst. In
fresh feces, oocysts of various species of coccidia may appear
similar to one another; however, once sporulation occurs, cocci-

---

Fecal Culture of Roundworm Eggs

Materials: glass jar with a tight-fitting cap
          wooden tongue depressors
          artist's paint brush
          Bunsen burner or alcohol burner

1) Place 20-30 g of the fresh fecal sample in a jar. Break up the feces with a tongue
depressor and moisten slightly with tap water. The mixture should not be so wet as
to appear "soupy."

2) Place the jar on a shelf away from direct sunlight and allow it to incubate at room
temperature for 7 days. There should be enough moisture so that droplets of
condensed water can be seen on the sides of the glass jar; if not, add a few drops
of water.

3) Some species of larvae can migrate up the walls of the jar. These may be
recovered by removing condensation drops off the glass with the paint brush and
transferring them to a drop of water on a microscope slide. Other species must be
recovered with the Baermann technique (see below).

4) Apply a coverslip to the slide (a drop of diluted Lugol's iodine may be added)
and pass it over the open flame of the Bunsen burner once or twice to kill the larvae
in an extended position. Place on the microscope slide stage and identify the larvae.

dia of the genus *Eimeria* can be easily distinguished from those of the genus *Isospora*. A fully sporulated oocyst of *Eimeria* contains 4 sporocysts, while a sporulated *Isospora* oocyst has 2 sporocysts (Fig 15).

Sample Collection at Necropsy

The postmortem examination (necropsy) is an important method for diagnosing parasitism of the digestive tract. Lesions of internal organs are often fairly indicative of the type of parasite that produced them. The veterinary technician is responsible for assisting during necropsy procedures and, in par-

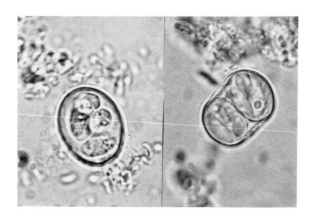

Figure 15. Fully sporated oocysts of *Eimeria* (left) and *Isospora* (right). (1400X)

Sporulation of Coccidial Oocysts

Materials: beakers or waxed paper cups
    Petri plates
    2.5% solution of potassium dichromate
    wooden tongue depressors
    materials for centrifugal flotation and sedimentation

1) When coccidia oocysts are found in a fresh fecal sample, place 10-20 g of the sample in a beaker or paper cup and cover with about 60 ml of 2.5% potassium dichromate solution. Mix thoroughly with a tongue depressor.

2) Pour into a Petri plate and allow to incubate at room temperature for 3-5 days. Open the plate daily and swirl the contents gently to allow air to reach the developing oocysts.

3) After incubation, centrifuge the plate's contents as described under the sedimentation procedure.

4) Process the fecal sediment by the centrifugal flotation procedure to recover the oocysts, which are then examined microscopically.

ticular, helping with preservation and processing of samples collected.

The contents of the digestive system may contain many types of parasites, some of which may be roundworms. Flukes and tapeworms are easily seen and can be individually isolated. The 2 preferred methods for recovering the roundworms are the decanting method and the sieving method. With either method, one should separate the contents of the different parts of the digestive tract into separate containers.

It is not always necessary to examine all sediment or sievings. An estimate of the number of worms may be obtained by counting an aliquot (a known percentage of the total volume) of the sediment.

When parasites are recovered from the digestive tract or other parts of the body, it may be necessary to preserve them for identification later. Roundworms should be briefly washed in water to remove any attached debris and then placed in hot 70% ethyl alcohol (ethanol). Isopropyl alcohol may be used but is not preferred. The alcohol is allowed to cool, after which the worms

---

Decanting Method

Materials: buckets large enough to hold the contents of each part of the digestive tract and an equal volume of water
knives
metal spatulas
stirring spoons or paddles
dissecting pans
dissecting microscope or magnifying glass
thumb forceps

1) Open each organ of the digestive tract and pour its contents into a bucket. Scrape the interior lining of the organ with the spatula or blunt edge of a pair of scissors and add the scrapings into the bucket or examine them separately.

2) Add an equal volume of water to the contents in each bucket and mix thoroughly with the spoon.

3) Allow the heavier part of the contents to settle to the bottom (usually about 45 minutes) and carefully pour off the liquid on top, leaving the sediment.

4) Add an equal volume of water to the sediment and stir. Allow this to resettle. Repeat this process until the water over the sediment becomes clear.

5) Pour off the clear water over the sediment, then transfer the sediment to the dissection pan.

6) Using the dissection microscope, examine a small amount of the sediment at a time. Any parasite found should be gently removed from the sediment with thumb forceps and preserved, as discussed later in this section.

Sieving Method

Materials: (materials as for decanting method)
  testing sieves, No. 18 (1.0-mm mesh) and No. 45 (0.354-mm mesh)
  (Sargent-Welch Scientific, Skokie, IL 60077)

1) Place the contents of each organ and the scrapings in a bucket and mix with water, as described for the decanting method.
2) Pour the mixture through the No. 18 sieve and then through the No. 45 sieve. Wash the sieves' contents with water.
3) Examine the material in the sieves, as described for the sediment in the decanting method.

---

are examined. The worms may be stored in the alcohol after adding glycerine to make a 5% concentration. Tapeworms, including the scolices (heads), should be placed in water at about 37 C (98.6 F) for about one hour and then stored in a mixture of 5% glycerin and 70% alcohol or 5-10% formalin. Flukes may be preserved like tapeworms. If tapeworms and flukes are to be stained later, they should be relaxed in alternate changes of ice water and tap water for about 3 hours and then lightly pressed between sheets of glass immersed in 10% formalin.

Sometimes during necropsy of domestic animals, "bladder worms" may be seen in the abdomen, muscles or internal organs. These are the larval stages of certain species of tapeworms and appear as fluid-filled, balloon-like structures that vary from the size of a pea up to the size of a basketball, depending on the species of tapeworm. Caution should be used in handling these parasites, as the fluid in them could be allergenic.

A discussion of identification of species of parasites recovered during necropsy is beyond the scope of this book. When specific identification is required, the technician may consult the references listed at the end of this chapter. Government or private diagnostic laboratories are useful in assisting with identification when questions arise, but they must be supplied with well-preserved specimens.

Shipping Parasitologic Specimens

Any parasite specimen shipped to a diagnostic laboratory by the US Postal Service or other carriers should be in a preservative, such as alcohol or formalin, to render it noninfectious. Specimens must be well packed so they do not leak; otherwise, the package may be refused for shipment.

Fecal materials should be mixed with 10% formalin at a ratio of 1 volume of feces to 3 volumes of formalin and placed in a screw-cap vial of 20- to 30-ml capacity. The vials should be sealed with tape and labeled with the practitioner's name, the client's name, and the species of animal, its name or number, sex and age. Worm specimens preserved in alcohol or formalin should be shipped in similar vials. The vials should be wrapped in absorbent material, such as toilet paper or paper towels, and placed in styrofoam mailing containers or heavy cardboard mailing tubes.

A cover letter should be sent to the diagnostic laboratory giving all pertinent information about the animal, a brief description of its clinical history and the diagnostic question requiring an answer.

Miscellaneous Procedures for Detection of Digestive Tract Parasites

Cellophane Tape Preparation

The cellophane tape preparation is used to detect the eggs of pinworms. Pinworms are a type of roundworm that protrudes out of the anus and deposits its eggs on the skin around the anus. Their eggs are usually not seen in routine fecal examinations.

Cellophane Tape Preparation

Materials: transparent adhesive (Scotch) tape
wooden tongue depressor
microscope slide

1) Place the tape in a loop around one end of the tongue depressor, with the adhesive side out.

2) Stand to the side of the horse's hindquarters and raise the tail with one hand while using the other hand to press the tape on the tongue depressor firmly against the skin immediately around the anus.

3) Place a small drop of water (or xylene) on the slide. Undo the loop of tape and stick it onto the slide, allowing the water to spread out under the tape.

4) Examine the tape microscopically for the presence of pinworm eggs (see Chapter 5).

Of the major domestic species, only horses are infected by pinworms (*Oxyuris equi*).

Baermann Technique

The Baermann technique is used to recover the larvae of roundworms from feces, soil or animal tissue. This method takes advantage of the fact that warm water stimulates the larvae in a sample to move about. Once the larvae move out of the sample, they relax in the water and sink to the bottom of the container. A Baermann apparatus must be constructed to perform this technique (Fig 16). The apparatus consists of a ring stand and a ring supporting a large funnel. The funnel's stem is connected by a piece of rubber tubing to a tapered tube (cut-off Pasteur pipette). The rubber tubing is clamped shut with a pinch clamp. A piece of metal screen is placed in the funnel to serve as a support for the sample. The funnel is then filled with water or physiologic saline at about 30 C (86 F) to a level 1-3 cm above the sample.

Larvae recovered from very fresh ruminant and equine feces are almost always lungworms. *Strongyloides* larvae may be found in canine feces. *Aelurostrongylus abstrusus*, the feline lungworm, may be recovered from the feces of cats.

Blood in the Feces

Some parasitic infections of the digestive tract cause extensive damage to the intestinal lining, resulting in bleeding. This

---

Baermann Technique

Materials: Baermann apparatus (as described above)
cheesecloth or gauze square about twice the diameter of the funnel
microscope slides and coverslips

1) Spread the cheesecloth out on the support screen in the Baermann apparatus. Take 5-15 g of the fecal, soil or tissue sample and place it on the cheesecloth. Fold any excess cheesecloth over the top of the sample. Be sure the sample is covered by the warm water or saline; add more if necessary.

2) Allow the apparatus to remain undisturbed overnight.

3) Hold a microscope slide under the cutoff pipette and open the pinch clamp only long enough to allow a large drop to fall on the slide. Apply a coverslip to the slide and examine it microscopically for larvae. Repeat by examining several slides before deciding the sample is negative.

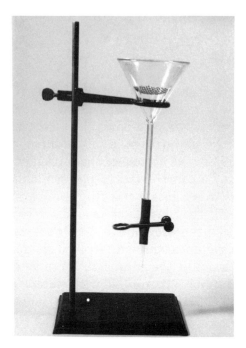

Figure 16. Baermann apparatus.

blood may be visible in the fecal sample or may be present in such small quantities that it is only detectable by means of a chemical test. Blood present in such small amounts is termed occult blood. Numerous tests are available for the detection of blood in feces. The simpler tests are based on detection of the enzyme-like activity of the RBC component, hemoglobin (*eg*, Hematest Reagent Tablets: Ames Division, Miles Laboratories, Elkhart, IN). These tests are easily performed by following the directions provided by the manufacturer. Blood is detected through an obvious color change. False-positive results may be obtained in samples from animals on a meat diet, so dogs and cats to be tested should be maintained on a meat-free diet for 24-48 hours before testing. Fecal blood may be present due to conditions other than parasitic infections, such as GI ulcers, other infectious agents and neoplasms.

Gross Examination of Vomitus

Vomitus (product of vomiting) may be grossly examined for adult parasites. These may be particularly common in the vomitus of puppies or kittens, in which infections with *Toxocara* or *Toxascaris* may be extensive and some of the worms are expelled by vomiting.

DIAGNOSIS OF PARASITISM
OF THE BLOOD AND VASCULAR SYSTEM

Dirofilaria immitis, the canine heartworm, is the most important parasite of the vascular system in domestic animals in the United States. For this reason, most of the blood examinations for parasites in veterinary practices are aimed specifically at heartworm identification, though some other blood parasites may be occasionally seen in the United States. This section describes some general tests that may be used to detect a number of blood parasites, as well as some specific tests for canine heartworms.

As mentioned in the section on parasites of the digestive tract, the technician must maintain a clean and orderly work area to perform effective diagnostic tests. Samples not properly labeled and results not immediately written down result in having to repeat tests, or may result in other complicating consequences.

Collection of Blood Samples

Any collection of blood from an animal should be performed aseptically. This includes swabbing the skin over the vein with alcohol and using a sterile needle.

Blood may be drawn with a syringe or a vacuum collection tube (*eg,* Vacutainer: Becton-Dickinson, Rutherford, NJ). No anticoagulant is required if the blood is to be used immediately for tests, such as the direct smear or filter test, or if it is to be allowed to clot so that serum may be obtained. If the tests cannot be performed immediately or if some of the blood must be retained for further testing, clotting must be prevented by addition of an anticoagulant.

Vacuum blood collection tubes are sold containing several different anticoagulants, with color-coded stoppers indicating the anticoagulant contained. Of these, ethylene diamine-tetraacetic acid (EDTA), in tubes with a lavender stopper, is among the best for collecting blood for parasite examination due to the minimum amount of distortion it produces. If the blood must be allowed to clot to obtain the clear serum, as for immunologic tests for canine heartworm, red-stopper vacuum tubes, which contain no anticoagulant, should be used.

Blood samples should always be labeled with the client's name, the animal's name or number, and the date of collection.

The microfilariae of *Dirofilaria immitis* are more common in canine blood at certain times of the day than at others. In the United States, the most microfilariae are found in blood samples obtained around 4:30 PM and the least around 11 AM.

Examination of Blood

General observations of blood samples should always be recorded. For example, if the blood appears watery, the animal may be anemic. Clinical pathology tests, such as packed cell volume and WBC counts, may aid in diagnosis of parasitism.

Direct Microscopic Examination

The simplest blood parasite detection procedure is by direct microscopic examination of whole blood. This procedure is aimed mainly at detecting movement of parasites that live outside of blood cells. In the United States, this is usually used to detect the microfilariae of the canine heartworm, *Dirofilaria immitis;* trypanosomes also may be seen. It is quick and easy to perform, but only a small amount of blood is examined. Unless the parasites are present in large numbers, they may be missed.

Trypanosomes are primarily found in tropical areas but may occasionally be found in the United States. They are more easily

---

Direct Microscopic Examination of Whole Blood

Materials: blood collection equipment
microscope slides and coverslips

1) Immediately after collecting the blood sample, place a single drop from the needle in the center of a slide and cover it with a coverslip.

2) Transfer the slide to a microscope stage and examine it systematically with 10X objective. Watch for localized areas of movement among blood cells, which may indicate the presence of parasites.

identified on stained blood smears (described below) than by direct examination of whole blood.

The microfilariae of primary interest in this country are those found in dogs, including microfilariae of *D immitis* and *Dipetalonema*. Differentiation between *Dirofilaria immitis* and *Dipetalonema* is very important, as the treatment for *D immitis* can be stressful and is unnecessary for dogs infected with *Dipetalonema*.

Direct microscopic examination of whole blood is a poor method for differentiating microfilariae, but there are some general rules that may be helpful. Usually the microfilariae of *D immitis* are more numerous than those of *Dipetalonema;* however, *D immitis* microfilariae may be seen in small numbers in some samples. Microfilariae of *Dipetalonema reconditum,* the most common species of *Dipetalonema* in the US, tend to move rapidly across the microscopic field with a snake-like movement. *Dirofilaria immitis* microfilariae tend to remain in one general area and coil and uncoil; however, in freshly drawn blood containing an anticoagulant, *D immitis* microfilariae may sluggishly move across the slide.

Thin Blood Smear

A thin blood smear is prepared in the same way as a blood smear prepared for a WBC differential count.

The area of the smear farthest from the original drop of blood should be the thinnest part of the smear (the "feathered edge"). Because of the large relative size of the microfilariae, they are carried to the feathered edge. A thin blood smear cannot be used for proper differentiation of *D immitis* from *Dipetalonema* microfilariae. Trypanosomes can be seen between the blood cells in the smear. Protozoa and rickettsiae, which live within or on blood cells, may be seen in thin blood smears.

The previous blood examination techniques used minute amounts of blood. Unless the parasites are present in large numbers, an infection may be missed. To be sure mild infections are not missed, several blood-concentration techniques using larger volumes of blood have been developed.

Figure 17. Demonstration of the correct angle and direction of movement for preparation of a thin blood smear.

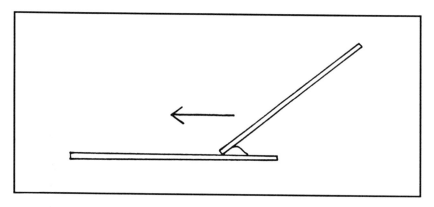

Thick Blood Smear

A thick blood smear allows examination of a slightly larger amount of blood than with a thin smear. Microfilariae, protozoa and rickettsiae may be seen using this method.

Buffy Coat Method

The buffy coat method is a concentration technique for detection of microfilariae in blood samples. The buffy coat is the layer of WBC located between the RBC and the clear plasma formed by centrifugation of whole blood. The specific gravity of micro-

---

Thin Blood Smear

Materials: microscope slides
blood smear fixative and stains (eg, Diff-Quik)

1) Place one slide flat on a bench and place a small drop of the blood sample near one end of the slide.

2) Place the end of a second slide near the middle of the first slide and hold it at a 45-degree angle. Holding the second slide at that angle, move the end of the second slide across the first slide until it just touches the drop of blood. Allow the blood to spread across the edge of the second slide.

3) Hold the first slide firmly against the bench. Push the second slide all the way across the first slide while applying firm, steady pressure (Fig 17). This forms a thin blood film across the face of the first slide.

4) Allow the slide to air dry and then stain it. Examine the slide with the 10X objective for microfilariae or trypanosomes and with the 100X objective (oil) for intracellular parasites.

Thick Blood Smear

Materials: microscope slides
distilled water
methyl alcohol
Giemsa stain (Harleco, Philadelphia, PA) diluted at 1:20 with
distilled water

1) Place 3 drops of the blood sample together on a slide and spread them out to an area about 2 cm in diameter.

2) Allow to air dry.

3) Place the slide in a slanted position, smear side down, in a beaker containing distilled water. Allow the slide to remain in the water until the smear loses its red color.

4) Remove and air dry the slide, then immerse it for 10 minutes in methyl alcohol. Stain with Giemsa stain for 30 minutes. Wash excess stain with tap water.

Buffy Coat Method

Materials: hematocrit (capillary) tubes and sealant
hematocrit centrifuge
small file or glass cutter
microscope slides and coverslips
physiologic saline
methylene blue stain (diluted 1:1000 with distilled water)

1) Fill the hematocrit tube with the blood sample and seal one end.

2) Centrifuge for 5 minutes.

3) Read the PCV of desired, then observe the location of the buffy coat, between the red cells and plasma (Fig 18).

4) Using the file, deeply scratch the glass at the level of the buffy coat. Snap the tube by applying thumb pressure opposite the scratch. Immediately take the part of the tube containing the buffy coat and plasma, and tap the buffy coat onto the center of a microscope slide, including some plasma with it.

5) Add a drop of saline and a drop of methylene blue stain, and cover with a coverslip. Examine the slide for microfilariae (Fig 19).

---

filariae causes them to gravitate to the upper surface of the buffy coat layer. The test is quick and can be done in conjunction with a packed cell volume (PCV); however, the species of microfilariae cannot be differentiated.

Modified Knott's Technique

The modified Knott's technique is a fairly rapid method that allows differentiation between *Dirofilaria immitis* and *Dipetalonema reconditum* microfilariae. It concentrates the micro-

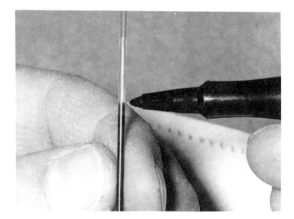

Figure 18. Buffy coat in a hematocrit tube.

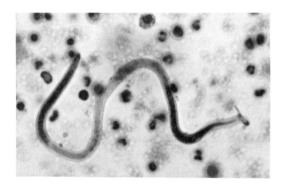

Figure 19. Microfilaria in a buffy coat smear of canine blood. (560X)

filariae from an adequate volume of blood and hemolyzes the RBC so microfilariae may be seen more clearly.

Using the modified Knott's technique, the characteristics in Table 1 can be used to distinguish *Dirofilaria immitis* from *Dipetalonema reconditum* microfilariae. These characteristics should not be used with other heartworm detection tests. The most accurate of the characteristics are body length, mid-body width and shape of the cranial end. Body length and width should be measured using a micrometer. The cranial end of *Dirofilaria immitis* microfilariae tapers gradually from mid-body, while *Dipetalonema reconditum* microfilariae have a blunt cranial end (Figs 20, 21). When using Table 1, observe as many

---

Modified Knott's Technique

Materials: 15-ml centrifuge tubes, with caps or stoppers
centrifuge
2% formalin (2 ml of 40% formaldehyde/98 ml distilled water)
methylene blue stain (diluted 1:1000 with distilled water)
Pasteur pipettes and pipette bulbs

1) Mix 1 ml of the blood sample and 9 ml of 2% formalin in a centrifuge tube. Stopper the tube and rock it back and forth for 1-2 minutes until the mixture becomes clear red (wine red).

2) Centrifuge the tube at 1500 rpm for 5 minutes.

3) Pour off the liquid supernatant, leaving the sediment at the bottom of the tube.

4) Add a drop of methylene blue stain to the sediment. Using a pipette, mix the sediment and stain. Transfer a drop of the mixture to a slide and apply a coverslip.

5) Examine the slide for microfilariae using the 10X microscope objective. When they are found, use a higher-power objective to differentiate them (Table 1).

---

microfilariae on the slide as possible before identifying them as *Dirofilaria immitis* or *Dipetalonema reconditum*.

Filter Technique

The filter technique is another means of concentrating microfilariae in blood samples. The materials required are available as diagnostic kits from various companies, including the Di-Fil Test Kit (Evsco) and the Heartworm Diagnostic Test Kit (Pitman-Moore). These kits contain complete directions for use. One ml of the blood sample (no anticoagulant is required if the test is performed immediately) is mixed with 9 ml of a blood cell lysing solution in a 10- or 12-ml syringe. A new, disposable, porous filter is placed in the filter holder. The fluid in the syringe is injected into the filter holder and is then flushed with 10 ml of water. Unlysed cells and microfilariae are retained on the surface of the filter. The filter is then gently transferred to a

Table 1. Characteristics for differentiation of microfilariae.

Characteristic	*Dirofilaria immitis*	*Dipetalonema reconditum*
Body shape	Usually straight	Usually curved
Body length	295-325 μ	250-288 μ
Midbody width	5-7.5 μ	4.5-5.5 μ
Shape of cranial end	Tapered	Blunt
Shape of tail	Straight	Usually curved or hooked

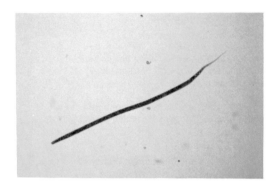

Figure 20. Microfilaria of *Dirofilaria immitis*, found using the modified Knott's technique. Note the straight tail and tapering cranial end. (225X)

microscope slide and stained with 2 drops of the stain included in the kit. The filter is covered with a coverslip and examined with a 10X objective for microfilariae (Fig 22).

The filter technique uses an amount of blood equal to that used in the modified Knott's technique and can be rapidly performed. Microfilarial species cannot be differentiated using the filter technique; therefore, if microfilariae are found, additional tests are required to determine if the infection is due to *D immitis* or *D reconditum*.

Immunologic Heartworm Tests

About 25% of dogs with adult heartworm infections in the heart do not have circulating microfilariae in the blood. The

Figure 21. Cranial (A) and caudal (B) ends of a microfilaria of *Dipetalonema reconditum*. (560X)

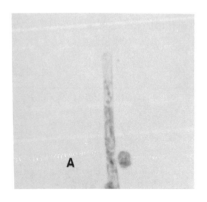
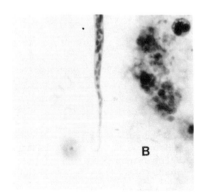

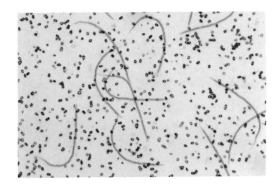

Figure 22. Microfilariae in canine blood on a filter. The small, irregular structures are the holes in the filter paper, while the small, circular structures are RBC. (140X)

infections may consist of worms too young to produce microfilariae, a unisex infection or infection in which circulating microfilariae have been killed by a drug but the adults have not been affected. This type of heartworm infection is referred to as an "occult infection." In addition, cats can be infected by canine heartworms. Because the worms are not in their natural host (dogs), in cats they shed low levels of microfilariae or none at all.

To detect infections, tests have been developed in which antibodies against antigens of adult *Dirofilaria immitis* react with a chemical to produce a color change when those antigens are in a blood sample. They are available commercially for use in practices from suppliers, including Uni-Tec CHW (Pitman-Moore, Mundelein, IL) and CITE Canine Heartworm Test Kit (IDEXX, Portland, ME). They are easy to perform and fairly rapid (15-20 minutes) if directions are carefully followed and good labeling of samples is maintained. Older-style kits detected only canine antibodies produced in response to heartworms and were unsuitable for use in cats.

Other tests for such parasites as *Toxoplasma gondii* can be performed by diagnostic labs. You should consult with the lab regarding the nature and amount of specimens they require. A method for collecting serum for these tests is described below.

Miscellaneous Methods

Other heartworm diagnostic procedures used in detection and differentiation of microfilariae include brilliant cresyl blue staining and acid phosphatase staining. These procedures are too cumbersome to be useful in a veterinary practice.

DIAGNOSIS OF PARASITISM OF THE RESPIRATORY SYSTEM

Fecal Examination for Respiratory Parasites

The life cycles of helminth parasites of the lungs are completed through passage of their eggs or larvae up the airways to the throat, from which they are swallowed and passed out in the feces. Because of this dependence on fecal transmission, parasitism of the lungs and airways is often diagnosed by microscopic examination of the feces as described previously.

Examination of Sputum and Tracheal Washes

The larvae and/or eggs of respiratory parasites found in the sputum or tracheal washes have the same characteristics as those found in the feces. An exception is *Dictyocaulus*, lungworms of cattle and sheep, which are usually seen as eggs containing larvae rather than as free larvae, as in the feces.

A drop of sputum or nasal discharge on a microscope slide is easily examined. Several slides should be examined. When the sputum is especially viscous, a drop of the material should be squashed between 2 microscope slides and both slides then

---

Serum Collection

Materials: needles and syringes
blood collection vacuum tubes without anticoagulant (red stopper), 16 x 100 mm (do not use plastic tubes)
applicator sticks

1) Collect 10 ml of blood for each tube to be submitted. Slowly dispense blood from the syringe into the tube to avoid lysis of RBC, which would interfere with the test.

2) Keep the blood at room temperature (25 C) for 2-3 hours to allow a solid clot to form.

3) Remove the clot with applicator sticks by gently "ringing" the clot (separating the clot from the glass) and then sliding it up the side of the tube while holding it between 2 sticks. Discard the clot. Some laboratories then request that the clear serum be transferred to a new tube.

4) Properly label each tube of serum with the client's name, animal's name or number, and the practitioner's name. Refrigerate the serum until it can be shipped.

5) Ship samples to the laboratory packed in an insulated container with ice by the fastest means available.

examined microscopically. Larger quantities of fluid obtained from the respiratory tract should be concentrated by centrifugation at 1500 rpm for 5 minutes. A drop of the sediment can then be placed on a slide and examined microscopically.

Dogs may occasionally become infested with the nasal mite, *Pneumonyssus caninum*. A cotton swab dipped in mineral oil may be inserted into the nose of a suspect dog and rubbed against the nasal membranes. The swab is then rubbed on a microscope slide. The mites have 8 legs, and are pale and 1-1.5 mm long.

DIAGNOSIS OF PARASITISM OF THE URINARY SYSTEM

Roundworms are common parasites of the kidney and urinary bladder. They complete their life cycles by passing their eggs out of the host's body in the urine. They include *Capillaria* spp, which inhabits the walls of the urinary bladder of dogs and cats, *Dioctophyma renale*, the giant kidney worm of dogs, and *Stephanurus dentatus*, the swine kidney worm.

Collection of the Urine Sample

Urine for parasitologic examination may be collected during normal urination. Catheterization is not necessary unless part of the sample is to be used for bacteriologic or cytologic examination. A waxed paper cup (3-5 fl oz) with lid or other clean container may be used for collection. The cup is held in the urine

---

Urine Sedimentation

Materials: 15-ml centrifuge tubes with conical tip
centrifuge
pipettes and bulb
microscope slides and coverslips

1) Thoroughly mix the urine sample and put 5-10 ml into a centrifuge tube.

2) Centrifuge the sample for 5 minutes at 1500 rpm.

3) Pipette all but about 0.5 ml of the fluid from the centrifuge tube, leaving the sediment at the bottom undisturbed.

4) Mix the remaining fluid and sediment together with the pipette; transfer a drop of this mixture to a microscope slide and apply a coverslip.

5) Thoroughly examine the drop of sediment microscopically, using the 10X objective.

stream and filled. Unless the sample is to be used for other tests, it is not necessary to collect the sample at a certain time during urination. Clients can collect a sample at home. Urine samples should be properly labeled with the client's name and the animal's identification, and refrigerated until the examination can be conducted.

Urine Examination for Parasites

The primary method of examining urine for parasites is by microscopic examination of the sediment.

DIAGNOSIS OF PARASITISM OF THE SKIN

L.P. Schmeitzel and P.J. Ihrke

Collection of Specimens

Skin Scrapings

The skin scraping is one of the most common diagnostic tools used in evaluating animals with dermatologic problems. Equipment needed includes an electric clipper with a #40 blade, a scalpel or spatula, mineral oil in a small dropper bottle, and a microscope. Typical lesions or sites likely to harbor the particular parasite should be scraped (eg, ear margins for *Sarcoptes scabiei*).

The scraping is performed with a #10 scalpel blade, used with or without a handle. A 165-mm stainless-steel spatula (Sargent-Welsh Scientific, Detroit) is preferred by some clinicians. The scalpel blade should be held between the thumb and second finger, with the first finger used to help prevent cutting the animal (Fig 23). Before the skin is scraped, the blade is dipped in a drop of mineral oil on the slide, or a drop of mineral oil may be placed on the skin.

During the scraping process, the blade must be held perpendicular to the skin. Holding it at another angle may result in an incision. The average area scraped should be 6-8 cm².

The depth of the scraping varies with the typical location of the parasite in question. When scraping for mites that live in burrows or hair follicles (eg, *Sarcoptes, Demodex*), the skin

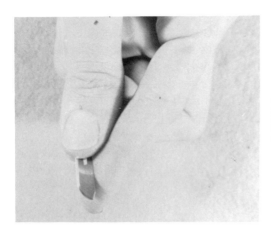

Figure 23. A safe method of holding a scalpel blade with the thumb and second finger for skin scrapings.

should be scraped until a small amount of capillary blood oozes from the area. Clipping the area with a #40 blade before scraping enables better visualization of the lesion and removes excess hair that impedes proper scraping and interferes with collection of epidermal debris. For surface-dwelling mites (eg, *Chorioptes, Cheyletiella*), the skin is scraped superficially to collect loose scales and crusts. Clipping before scraping is not always necessary when infestation with surface dwellers is suspected.

All of the scraped debris on the forward surface of the blade is then spread in a drop of mineral oil on a slide. A glass coverslip is placed on the material and the slide is ready for microscopic examination using the 4X (scanner) objective. The slide should be examined systematically in rows so the entire area under the coverslip is evaluated (Fig 8). Low light intensity and high contrast increase visualization of translucent mites and eggs. If necessary, the slide may be evaluated using the 10X (low power) objective.

Demonstration of a characteristic mite or egg is frequently diagnostic for most diseases. In certain circumstances, more than just identification of the parasite is necessary. For example, determining live:dead ratios and observing immature stages of demodectic mites are important in evaluating a patient with demodicosis. A decrease in the number of live mites and eggs during therapy is a good prognostic sign.

Cellophane-Tape Preparation

When attempting to demonstrate the presence of lice or mites that live primarily on the surface of the skin (*eg, Cheyletiella*), a cellophane-tape preparation may be used instead of a skin scraping. Clear cellophane tape (Scotch Transparent Tape: 3M) is applied to the skin to pick up epidermal debris. A ribbon of mineral oil is placed on a glass slide and the adhesive surface of the tape is then placed on the mineral oil. Additional mineral oil and a coverslip may be placed on the tape to prevent the tape from wrinkling, but this is not necessary. The slide is then examined for parasites.

DIAGNOSIS OF PARASITISM OF MISCELLANEOUS BODY SYSTEMS

W.F. Wade and S.M. Gaafar

Parasites of the Eye

Thelazia are roundworms that live on the eyes of several species of domestic animals, including cattle, sheep, goats, horses, dogs and cats. The adult parasites are milky white and 7-17 mm long, and reside under the eyelids, particularly the third eyelid, and on the surface of the eyeball. Diagnosis is made by anesthetizing the eye with a local ophthalmologic anesthetic and directly examining the eye for parasites.

Parasites of the Ear

Otodectes cynotis, the ear mite, is a very common cause of external ear irritation in dogs and cats. These white mites are frequently seen during otoscopic examination. They may also be seen by using a cotton swab moistened with mineral oil to remove some of the dark, waxy debris found in the ears of infested animals. This material is transferred to a drop of mineral oil on a microscope slide and spread out with the swab. A coverslip is applied to the debris and the slide is examined microscopically (Fig 24).

Parasites of the Genital Tract

Tritrichomonas foetus is a protozoan parasite of the reproductive tract of cattle. They reside in the prepuce of infected bulls

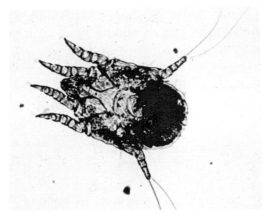

Figure 24. *Otodectes cynotis* from the ear of a dog. (120X)

and the vagina, cervix and uterus of infected cows. *Tritricho-monas foetus* is pear shaped and 10-25 μ long, with a sail-like membrane and 3 rapidly moving, whip-like flagellae on its cranial end (Fig 25). In fresh specimens they move actively with a jerky motion. Diagnosis is by finding the organisms in fluid collected from the stomach of an aborted fetus, uterine discharges or washings of the vagina and prepuce (Fig 26). Fluid material should be centrifuged at 2000 rpm for 5 minutes. The supernatant is then removed and a drop of the sediment transferred to a slide for microscopic examination for the organisms.

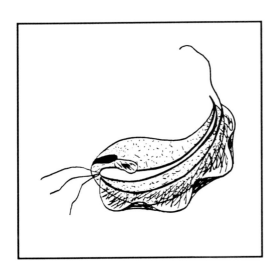

Figure 25. Diagram of *Tritrich-omonas foetus*. (6000X)

Several slides should be examined. For more accurate diagnosis, fluid material from the sources mentioned above can be cultured in special media. Specialized laboratories should be consulted for information on these techniques.

Figure 26. Appearance of tritrichomonads in a preputial smear from a bull.

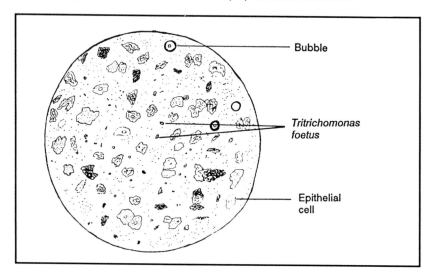

3

Internal Parasites of Dogs and Cats

C.A. St. Jean and L.A. Capitini

Roundworms

Roundworms or ascarids are one of the most common parasites found in puppies and kittens. The large roundworm of dogs is *Toxocara canis*; the large roundworm of cats is *Toxocara cati (Toxocara mystax)*. A less common ascarid, the roundworm of dogs and cats, is *Toxascaris leonina*. Adult roundworms inhabit the small intestine of their respective hosts.

Toxocara canis

Toxocara canis is the largest ascarid of dogs. Female adults measure over 20 cm long, while male adults are smaller, measuring around 10 cm long. These are long, white, straight worms, in contrast to the stomach worms of *Physaloptera* species, which are similar in size but C-shaped or curved. Clients may say *Toxocara canis* worms look a little like spaghetti (Chapter 2, Fig 5).

The eggs are unsegmented when passed in the feces, have a thick, pitted shell, and measure 90 x 75 μ (Fig 1). They are very resistant to adverse environmental conditions, and can survive on soil for several years. Under ideal conditions, eggs take about 2 weeks to embryonate and become infective.

Life Cycle: The life cycle of *Toxocara canis* is very interesting and rather complex. The 4 methods of transmission are direct, transplacental, transmammary and predation of paratenic hosts. Direct transmission by ingestion of the infective embryonated eggs leads to release of larvae in the intestinal tract, and migration to the liver and then to the lungs. This route is called hepatotracheal migration. These larvae migrate from the lungs, up the trachea, where they are swallowed. They molt to the adult stage, and eggs appear in the feces about one month after infection. The life span of these adults is about 4 months. Older dogs usually have larvae migrate though the circulatory system into various tissues and organs, especially muscle and kidney. This process is called somatic migration.

Transplacental transmission is the primary route of infection for puppies. Larvae in the tissues of the pregnant bitch become activated and migrate into the fetal liver, beginning about day 42 of gestation. Eggs can appear in the feces at 21 days of age in puppies infected prenatally. Why larvae become activated in pregnant bitches remains unclear, but it may be associated with changes in the immune state of the bitch.

Transmammary transmission occurs when larvae in the tissues and ingested infectious larvae pass in the bitch's milk to nursing puppies. These larvae develop directly to adult worms in the intestinal tract of the puppy. This route is a relatively

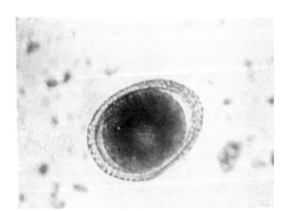

Figure 1. *Toxocara canis* egg. (400X)

unimportant method of infection, as most larvae are transmitted to puppies by the transplacental route.

The fourth mechanism of infection is by ingestion of paratenic hosts harboring infective larvae. Many animals can serve as paratenic hosts, including rodents, rabbits, earthworms, birds and flies. This mechanism is probably unimportant in dogs, but may be more important in predatory hosts, such as foxes.

Clinical Signs: Clinical signs of roundworm infection vary according to the number of parasites and the age of the dog. Some infected dogs have no signs, while heavily infected neonatal puppies may die. Common signs in puppies include unthriftiness, a pot-bellied appearance, dull haircoat, diarrhea or constipation, and possibly anemia.

Diagnosis: Toxocara canis infection is diagnosed by finding adult worms in the feces or vomitus (Chapter 2, Fig 5), and/or by performing a fecal flotation and finding the characteristic subglobular unsegmented eggs (Fig 1). Prepatent infections are diagnosed by clinical signs of listlessness, dull haircoat, coughing and distended abdomen, and the history of anthelmintic use.

Toxocara cati

Toxocara cati (T mystax) is the common roundworm of cats. Adult worms found in the small intestine of cats are smaller than the adult *Toxocara canis* worms of dogs. Adult male worms are about 6 cm long, while the larger adult females are about 12 cm long. Eggs of *Toxocara cati* are similar to those of *Toxocara canis* but are slightly smaller. They are unsegmented and almost spherical, with a pitted shell, and measure about 75 x 65 μ (Fig 2). Like *Toxocara canis* eggs, under ideal conditions the eggs of *Toxocara cati* become infective in about one month.

Life Cycle: The life cycle is similar to that of *Toxocara canis*, but the transplacental route of infection does not occur. The transmammary route is probably the main source of infection for kittens. Direct transmission by ingestion of infective eggs and by ingestion of paratenic hosts harboring larvae are other mechanisms of infection. Predation of paratenic hosts is more important in cats than in dogs. Ingestion of infectious eggs

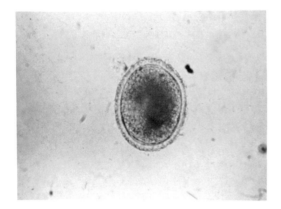

Figure 2. *Toxocara cati (mystax)* egg. (400X)

results in adult parasites in the intestine one month later. Eggs pass in the feces about 2 months later.

Ascarid infections in kittens are usually asymptomatic. More severe infections may cause a pot-bellied appearance, coughing, dull haircoat, vomiting, and diarrhea or constipation.

Diagnosis: Ascarid infection in cats is diagnosed by finding the adult worms in the feces or vomitus, and/or by performing a fecal flotation and finding the characteristic unsegmented, almost spherical eggs (Fig 2). Prepatent infections are diagnosed by clinical signs and the history of anthelmintic use.

Toxascaris leonina

Toxascaris leonina is the roundworm of dogs and cats. Adult worms are found in the small intestine. This worm is much less common than *Toxocara* species, and mixed infections of ascarids are rare. Adult *Toxascaris leonina* worms are slightly smaller than adult *Toxocara cati* worms. The eggs of *Toxascaris leonina* are different than those of *Toxocara* species (Fig 3). It is important to differentiate these eggs from those of *Toxocara* species because *Toxascaris leonina* is not a public health concern, while *Toxocara canis* and *Toxocara cati* have zoonotic potential.

Life Cycle: The life cycle of *Toxascaris leonina* is much less complex than that of *Toxocara* ascarids. Only 2 mechanisms of transmission occur with this parasite, direct transmission or ingestion of a paratenic host. Transplacental and transmammary transmission do not occur in infected cats or dogs.

The most common method of infection is by ingestion of infective eggs. Under optimal conditions, eggs embryonate and become infective in one week. After ingestion, the eggs hatch and larvae migrate into the intestinal wall. These larvae molt twice and develop into adults in the intestinal tract lumen. Hepatotracheal migration does not occur with this ascarid. The prepatent period is about 2 months.

Infection by ingestion of paratenic hosts also occurs. Mice, rabbits and chickens have been documented as paratenic hosts. *Toxascaris* infection does not appear to produce immunity, as *Toxocara* infection does. This parasite can therefore be found in adult dogs and cats. In contrast, *Toxocara canis* is considered to primarily infect young puppies, and is only occasionally found in adult dogs.

Toxascaris leonina appears to be the least pathogenic ascarid. The limited migration and lack of transmammary and transplacental transmission are important factors limiting pathogenicity. Infected cats and dogs usually have no clinical signs. Puppies

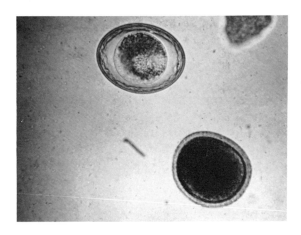

Figure 3. Eggs of *Toxascaris leonina* (top left) and *Toxocara canis* (lower right). (400X)

with severe infections may exhibit abdominal pain, vomiting, diarrhea, and occasionally death.

Diagnosis: Toxascaris leonina infection is diagnosed by fecal flotation and finding the characteristic ellipsoid eggs (Fig 3). The shell is thick and smooth on the outside, while the interior of the shell is very irregular. In fresh feces the centrally located nucleus is unsegmented and produces a halo appearance.

Public Health Significance

Only *Toxocara canis* and *Toxocara cati* have zoonotic potential through ingestion of infective eggs. *Toxascaris leonina* does not infect people. In children, ingestion of *T canis* or *T cati* eggs may lead to a condition called visceral larva migrans. Larvae migrate through the body, including the liver and lungs, and occasionally, the central nervous system and eyes. Blindness caused by larval invasion of the retina can be a serious problem in infected children. For this reason, the veterinarian and technician have an obligation to properly educate clients concerning prevention and elimination of ascarid infection in dogs and cats, and the public health significance of the *Toxocara* species.

Hookworms

Hookworms are very common parasites of young and adult dogs and cats. Two genera of hookworms in dogs and cats are *Ancylostoma* and *Uncinaria. Uncinaria* is more common in the northern United States and Canada, while *Ancylostoma* is more common in warmer climates.

Ancylostoma

The more common *Ancylostoma* species include *Ancylostoma caninum,* common dog hookworm; *Ancylostoma tubaeforme,* common cat hookworm; and *Ancylostoma braziliense,* hookworm of dogs and cats found in southern states. Adult worms are reddish brown and 6-20 mm long. Adult female worms are larger than the adult males.

Life Cycle: The life cycle of hookworms is direct. Transmission is by ingestion, percutaneous penetration, or transplacental or transmammary passage of the infective larvae. Regardless of the method of transmission, the prepatent period is about 2 weeks.

In direct transmission, segmented eggs passed in feces readily release the first-stage larvae in 24-48 hours, but this can take as few as 2 hours under ideal conditions. Third-stage infective larvae rapidly develop and are free living until they are ingested by a suitable definitive host. After they are ingested, larvae further develop in the small intestine, until fifth-stage larvae attach to the intestinal wall, mature to adults and produce eggs. The role of any somatic migration in oral ingestion is unknown.

In percutaneous infection, larvae penetrate the skin and migrate through the circulatory system into the lungs, trachea, esophagus, stomach and finally the small intestine, where the larvae mature into adult hookworms.

Some larvae may undergo somatic migration and encyst in skeletal muscle in a dormant stage for prolonged periods. Larvae in a stage of developmental rest are called hypobiotic larvae. Pregnancy activates these dormant larvae, and they subsequently migrate across the placenta into the fetus (transplacental transmission).

Larvae are also transmitted via the milk (transmammary transmission). Transmammary transmission varies among species, but this route appears to be the primary method of *Ancylostoma caninum* infection in puppies.

Clinical Signs: Clinical signs, if any, caused by cutaneous penetration through the skin depend upon the number of larvae, site of penetration, and the host's immune response. Most lesions occur in the interdigital skin and on the footpads, and appear as erythematous, superficially traumatized areas.

More common clinical signs are related to internal complications from the larvae and adults. Hookworms feed on blood and change feeding sites often. Excessive bleeding from the previous site of attachment produces profound anemia and protein loss. Classic hookworm disease manifests itself as iron deficiency anemia. Signs include lethargy, anorexia, dull haircoat, pale mucous membranes and tarry stool. Death from hookworm infection is common in untreated puppies.

Uncinaria stenocephala

The hookworm *Uncinaria stenocephala* is similar in size, life cycle, clinical signs and treatment to *Ancylostoma;* however, this parasite is found in the northern United States and Canada and is commonly known as the northern hookworm. Its eggs are similar to those of *Ancylostoma caninum* but are larger (Fig 4). Transmammary infection by *Uncinaria stenocephala* larvae can cause profound anemia and death of puppies within 12 days after birth.

Diagnosis: Hookworm infection is diagnosed by fecal flotation and finding the characteristic hookworm or strongyle-type eggs. These are elongated ellipsoid eggs with a smooth cell wall enclosing a segmented nucleus that contains 2-8 cells (Fig 4). This stage may be referred to as the morula stage. Eggs range in size from 56-65 x 37-43 μ for *Ancylostoma caninum* and *Ancylostoma tubaeforme,* to 65-80 x 40-50 μ for *Uncinaria stenocephala* (Fig 4).

Note that the eggs of *Ancylostoma braziliense* are similar in size to those of *Uncinaria stenocephala,* which are larger than the typical *Ancylostoma caninum* eggs. The species of hookworm present cannot be determined by measuring the eggs. Also, the number of eggs observed does not necessarily indicate the severity of the infection, though in puppies, the presence of any hookworm eggs should be considered serious.

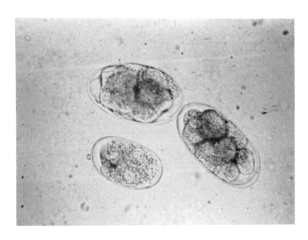

Figure 4. Different-sized hookworm eggs, possibly *Uncinaria stenocephala* (larger) eggs with an *Ancylostoma caninum* (smaller) egg.

Public Health Significance

Hookworms, especially *Ancylostoma braziliense*, cause cutaneous larva migrans in people. This condition is more prevalent in southern states.

Whipworms

Trichuris

Whipworms are common parasites of young and adult dogs. The common whipworm of dogs is *Trichuris vulpis*. Whipworms are very rare in cats. Two species of whipworms occasionally reported in cats are *Trichuris campanula* and *Trichuris serrata*. Most whipworm-type eggs found in cat feces are diagnosed as *Capillaria* eggs. These eggs can also be those of spurious parasites in mice, rabbits and birds eaten by cats. Adult whipworms are found in the cecum and large intestine of the definitive hosts.

Adult whipworms are 45-75 mm long. They are called whipworms because the long thin cranial end and the short thick caudal end give these worms a whip-like appearance. The characteristic whipworm egg is shaped like a lemon or football and has a thick smooth shell with an operculum at each end (Fig 5). These yellow-brown eggs are bilaterally symmetric and unembryonated in fresh feces. *Trichuris vulpis* eggs measure 70-89 x 37-40 μ. They are very resistant in the environment and may remain viable for years in the soil.

Life Cycle: The life cycle of whipworms is direct. Adult female worms produce unembryonated eggs that are passed in the feces. Under ideal conditions, these eggs embryonate and become infective in about 2 weeks. After ingestion by a suitable host, larvae emerge through the polar opercula of the egg. Larvae undergo several molts in the small and large intestine before attaching to the wall of the cecum or large intestine and developing into adults. The prepatent period for *Trichuris vulpis* is about 3 months (70-107 days); the adult life span varies between 5 and 16 months.

Clinical Signs: Clinical signs are usually mild in most whipworm infections. In young puppies, signs may include diarrhea, emaciation, dehydration, anemia and, in severe infections,

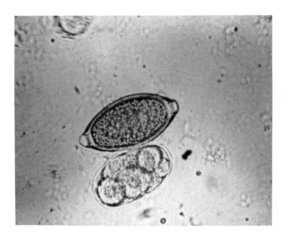

Figure 5. *Trichuris vulpis* (top) and *Ancylostoma caninum* (bottom) eggs. (400X)

death. In older dogs, the most common clinical sign is intermittent diarrhea containing mucus and fresh blood. Biting at the flank is a rarely reported clinical sign.

Diagnosis: Whipworm infection is diagnosed by fecal flotation and identifying the characteristic symmetric, unembryonated, thick-shelled, lemon-shaped egg with opercula at both ends (Fig 5). Dogs with frank signs of whipworm infection often have negative fecal examinations. Veterinarians usually treat these dogs for whipworms and wait to see if the signs abate. Fiberoptic endoscopes can be used in these dogs to make the diagnosis, but routine treatment is probably the preferred method. Because reinfection is possible, dogs should be rechecked at 3-month intervals.

Public Health Significance: Whipworms have been documented as a public health problem in Russia. Documentation in the United States is unclear. Discussion of proper waste management and hygiene with dog owners with small children at home is recommended.

Threadworms

Strongyloides

Strongyloides stercoralis is called the intestinal threadworm of people, dogs, foxes and cats. Another threadworm, *Strongy-*

loides tumefaciens, has been associated with tumors in the large intestine of cats.[1] These parasites are more commonly found in tropical climates, but they may also be present in temperate regions throughout the world. Only parthenogenetic female worms parasitize the intestinal tract of susceptible definitive hosts. The small adult female worms are about 2 mm long.

Life Cycle: The life cycle of *Strongyloides* is very unusual in that it includes separate parasitic and nonparasitic generations. Pathogenic female *Strongyloides* adults in the small intestine produce small embryonated eggs that pass in the feces. The exception to this is *Strongyloides stercoralis,* whose eggs hatch immediately in the intestinal tract, and first-stage larvae are found in the feces.

First-stage larvae in the soil can develop along 2 pathways: the homogonic cycle, in which first-stage larvae continue to develop into infective third-stage larvae; or the free-living cycle, in which first-stage larvae develop into nonparasitic male and female nematodes that produce larvae eventually developing into infective third-stage larvae. Note that free-living nematodes produce only infective larvae. Transmission is primarily by skin penetration.

Clinical Signs: The predominant clinical sign observed in dogs and cats infected with *Strongyloides* is intractable diarrhea. Skin penetration by infective larvae may cause intense pruritus, and migration through the lungs may cause verminous pneumonia. *Strongyloides stercoralis* infection can be a serious problem in young puppies.

Diagnosis: Intestinal threadworm infection is diagnosed by fecal smears and flotations. Flotations may distort the larvae, making differentiation difficult (Fig 6). Direct fecal smears are best for identifying the first-stage rhabditiform larvae of *Strongyloides stercoralis.* The fecal sample should be as fresh as possible. A fecal loop or a glove can be used to obtain fresh samples directly from the rectum for preparing smears. In dogs, first-stage rhabditiform larvae must be differentiated from the larvae of *Ancylostoma.*

Figure 6. A larva of *Strongy-loides stercoralis* from canine feces, as seen after flotation in a concentrated sugar solution. (140X)

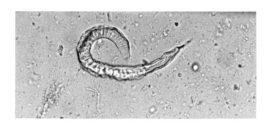

In cats, *Strongyloides tumefaciens* eggs contain a fully developed larva. This embryonated egg measures 114-124 x 62-68 μ. Fresh cat feces should be examined, and threadworm larvae must be differentiated from those of *Aelurostrongylus abstrusus*, the lungworm of cats. *Aelurostrongylus* larvae have a characteristically kinked tail (Fig 7).

The Baermann apparatus may also be used to establish a diagnosis. After incubation, the unique filariform infective larvae develop. All fecal samples, especially those suspected to contain *Strongyloides* larvae, should be handled properly to prevent contamination. Feces sent to a laboratory should be shipped in 10% formalin or 70% ethanol to preserve the larvae.

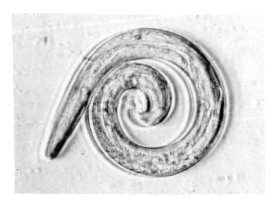

Figure 7. A larva of *Aelurostrongylus abstrusus* from feline feces. (560X)

Public Health Significance

Strongyloides stercoralis may cause disease in people, the severity depending on the pathogenicity of the strain involved. Good hygiene should be practiced to prevent infection in people.

Lungworms

Capillaria aerophila

Capillaria aerophila, sometimes called the fox lungworm, is found in the trachea and bronchi of dogs, cats and foxes. The eggs resemble those of *Trichuris* but are smaller and usually asymmetric (Fig 8). They measure 59-80 x 30-40 μ.

Diagnosis is made by finding the eggs in feces, bronchial secretions or nasal secretions. In dog and cat infections, clinical signs are uncommon. If signs develop, the main one is a chronic harsh cough. The life cycle is direct, and infective larvae develop in the eggs after 2 weeks. Ingestion of the infective embryonated eggs results in development of adults in the trachea and bronchi of suitable definitive hosts.

Filaroides osleri

Unlike the metastrongyloides, the lungworms *Filaroides osleri* and *Filaroides hirthi* have first-stage larvae that are directly

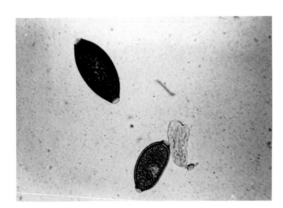

Figure 8. Symmetric *Trichuris* egg (top left) and an asymmetric smaller *Capillaria* egg (bottom right).

infective, and do not require an intermediate host.[2,3] Adult worms are found in the bronchi and trachea, where they form nodules. Larval stages develop in the lung and first-stage larvae pass into the saliva and feces. Infection is by ingestion of feces or lung tissue from infected dogs, or from an infected bitch grooming her puppies.

The prepatent period for *Filaroides osleri* is about 10 weeks and for *Filaroides hirthi* about 5 weeks. Clinical signs vary from persistent harsh dry cough in the usual chronic infection, to dypsnea and death. This parasite is uncommon in the United States, and infection is usually acquired early by young puppies.

Filaroides infection is diagnosed by finding the larvae in the sputum or feces. The Baermann technique for collecting larvae is not successful with *Filaroides osleri* and *Filaroides hirthi* because the larvae are not very active and do not escape from the fecal mass. Zinc sulfate flotation is more effective for finding *Filaroides* larvae, but bronchoscopic examination for nodule formation at the bifurcation of the trachea is the most reliable diagnostic procedure. *Filaroides osleri* is difficult to eradicate.

Aelurostrongylus abstrusus

Aelurostrongylus abstrusus is the common cat lungworm. Oviparous female adults lay unsegmented eggs in lung tissue. First-stage larvae are carried up the trachea and swallowed, and pass in the feces. These larvae have a characteristic kinked tail, and are very motile and readily demonstrated by the Baermann technique (Fig 7).

The life cycle is indirect. First-stage larvae must be ingested by a slug or snail. These intermediate hosts are probably ingested by paratenic hosts, which in turn are ingested by the definitive host, the cat. Adult worms develop in cats after the paratenic host is ingested, and larvae appear in the feces 5-6 weeks later.

Infected cats are often asymptomatic. Moderate infections may produce some coughing, while severe infections cause dyspnea, polypnea and possibly death. Levamisole has been used as treatment.

Bladder Worms

Capillaria

Capillaria plica is the common bladder worm of dogs, cats and foxes. Adult worms are 15-60 mm long, and females are larger than males. Adult worms are found in the urinary bladder and are considered nonpathogenic. No treatment is required. The life cycle is indirect, with earthworms acting as the intermediate hosts. Diagnosis is by finding the characteristic eggs in urine sediment (Fig 9). Eggs of *Capillaria felis cati* are similar and may appear in the urine of infected cats.[4]

Giant Kidney Worms

Dioctophyma

Dioctophyma renale is the largest known nematode. The giant kidney worm is found in the kidneys of dogs, foxes, otters, mink, weasels and wild carnivores. Larvae have been found in subcutaneous nodules in people. Male adults measure 35 cm, while female adults reach lengths up to 103 cm. Eggs are barrel shaped, with an operculum at both poles (Fig 10). The thick shell is pitted. The unsegmented eggs are brownish-yellow, measure 71-84 x 46-52 μ, and found in urine sediment.

The life cycle of *Dioctophyma renale* is indirect. The free-living worm, *Lumbriculus variegatus,* is the only intermediate host required to complete the life cycle. Paratenic hosts are probably

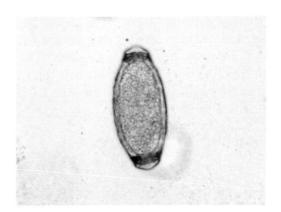

Figure 9. An egg of *Capillaria plica* from canine urine sediment. (350X)

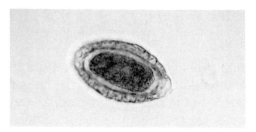

Figure 10. *Dioctophyma renale* egg in canine urine.

important in this life cycle also. Mink are the principal definitive hosts. The prepatent period in mink is almost 5 months.

Clinical signs range from asymptomatic to nervousness, emaciation, urine retention and death. Diagnosis is by demonstrating eggs in the urine. The only treatment is surgical removal of the worms from the kidney.

Esophageal Worms

Spirocerca lupi

Spirocerca lupi, also called the esophageal worm, is found in the esophagus of dogs, foxes, wolves and wild Felidae, such as lynx and snow leopards. Adult males are up to 54 mm long, while adult females are up to 80 mm long. The small thick-shelled, embryonated eggs are 30-37 x 11-15 μ. The life cycle of *Spirocerca lupi* is indirect. Beetles are the intermediate host. The definitive host may ingest a beetle or a paratenic host containing an infective larvae. These larvae migrates through the stomach wall into the circulatory system and eventually into the esophagus, where they form a large cellular mass. This mass may interfere with swallowing, and cause vomiting and emaciaton. The prepatent period of *Spirocerca lupi* is 5-6 months. This worm is the only parasite thought to be associated with tumor formation. Most cases of malignant esophageal sarcomas are related to *Spirocerca lupi* infections.[1]

Stomach Worms

Physaloptera

Physaloptera preputialis is the stomach worm of cats and *Physaloptera rara* is the stomach worm of dogs. Adult worms may be similar in size to adult ascarids. *Physaloptera* worms are C-shaped, while ascarids are straight. *Physaloptera* eggs are small, have a thick shell, and contain larvae (Fig 11).

The life cycle is indirect; beetles are a common intermediate host. Paratenic hosts probably have some importance in this life cycle. Adult worms attach to the stomach wall and suck blood. Clinical signs include vomiting, anorexia, and dark tarry stools. Diagnosis is by finding eggs in the feces. Eggs of *Physaloptera* must be differentiated from those of *Spirocerca lupi*.

Eyeworms

Thelazia californiensis

Thelazia californiensis is the eyeworm of sheep, deer, cattle, cats, dogs and people in the United States. These small worms are found in the conjunctival sac or tear duct of definitive hosts. The life cycle is indirect; various species of flies are the common intermediate hosts. Diagnosis is by finding the worms in the conjunctival sac, or by finding the embryonated egg or first-stage larvae in the tears. *Thelazia californiensis* causes conjunctivitis, pain and excessive lacrimation in people.

Heartworms

Dirofilaria immitis

Dirofilaria immitis is the heartworm of dogs. Canine heartworm disease is a major problem in many areas of the United

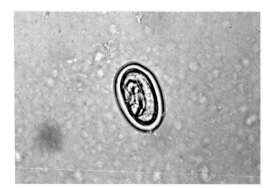

Figure 11. Egg of *Physaloptera rara*. (350X)

States. The nematode, *Dirofilaria immitis,* is transmitted by many species of mosquitoes to the principal host, the dog. Other hosts include cats, people and horses.

Adult heartworms are long, slender nematodes with cylindric bodies and thick cuticles. Male worms are smaller than the female worms, which are about 25 cm long. Though immature and adult worms are occasionally found in aberrant sites in the body, adult worms are usually found in the right ventricle and the pulmonary artery (Fig 12). Heartworms may also be found in the caudal vena cava and the right atrium.

Life Cycle: Knowledge of the life cycle of *Dirofilaria immitis* is important when explaining the diagnosis, treatment and prevention of heartworm infection to clients. Adult female heartworms produce first-stage larvae or microfilariae that circulate in the peripheral blood (Chapter 2, Figs 19, 20).

Microfilariae in the peripheral blood enter a mosquito when it bites the dog for a blood meal. In the mosquito, the micro-

Figure 12. Adult heartworms in the heart of a dog, as seen at necropsy.

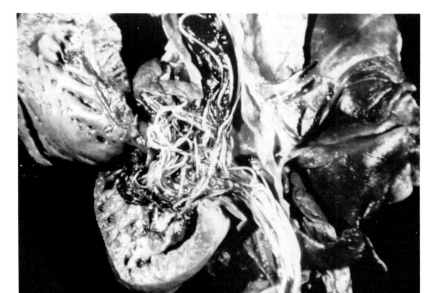

filariae develop to third-stage larvae and migrate to the mouth-parts of the mosquito. This period of development within the mosquito takes about 2 weeks.

When the mosquito bites another dog (or the same dog), the third-stage larvae enter the dog's body and migrate to the heart. At 4-5 months after infection (bite of infected mosquito), the larvae appear in the heart. Here they mature to adults, mate and produce microfilariae. These microfilariae begin appearing in peripheral blood 6-7 months after infection. Microfilariae that appear in the peripheral blood of puppies less than 6 months old are thought to be a result of prenatal infection from an infected bitch.

Diagnosis: Chapter 2 contains a discussion of diagnosis of heartworm infection.

Common reasons for false positive misdiagnosis when using the filter technique (see Chapter 2) include improperly cleaned filter holder, test tubes or syringes, and contaminated lysing solution. Washing and rinsing all equipment well after each test is an important step in preventing contamination from a previous positive test.

False positives from contamination of the lysing solution are probably more common. Some lysing solution containers are designed for aspirating the solution directly into the syringe containing the blood sample. The containers do not have a valve that prevents blood from being aspirated back into the stock reagent bottle. An efficient, economical alternative method is to prefill individual disposable pill containers with 10 ml of lysing solution for each sample being run. The lysing solution can then be readily aspirated form the individual pill container without contaminating the stock reagent in the bottle.

Reasons for obtaining false-negative results are using a filter with a pore size greater than 8 μ or using a wrinkled filter. Be certain to order the proper filters. More important, handle filters carefully and position filters carefully so the filter is not wrinkled or improperly positioned in the filter holder when the holder is assembled.

Once microfilariae are detected, they must be microscopically examined to determine if they are those of *Dirofilaria immitis* or of *Dipetalonema reconditum* (see Chapter 2).

Subcutaneous Worms

Dipetalonema reconditum

Dipetalonema reconditum is the subcutaneous worm of dogs. Adult male worms are up to 32 mm long, while females are up to 23 mm long. The life cycle of this parasite is indirect. Fleas (*Ctenocephalides* and *Pulex irritans*) and ticks (*Rhipicephalus sanguineus* and *Heterodoxus spiniger*) act as intermediate hosts. Infective larvae develop in the flea in one week; the prepatent period is about 9 weeks.

Dipetalonema reconditum is nonpathogenic, but microfilariae of *Dipetalonema* must be differentiated from those of *Dirofilaria immitis* (see Chapter 2).

Tapeworms

Dipylidium caninum

Dipylidium caninum is the flea tapeworm of dogs and cats. Tapeworms consist of a head (scolex) and numerous segments (proglottids), in a long flat shape that gives the worms their name. Tapeworms can be up to 50 cm long, and segments are often seen in the feces by clients (Chapter 2, Fig 2).

The life cycle is indirect, and the intermediate hosts are fleas (*Ctenocephalides*) and biting lice (*Trichodectes canis*) (Fig 13). After ingestion of the cysticercus located in the intermediate host, segment-shedding tapeworms develop in 2-3 weeks. Because of this short maturation period, control involves elimination of fleas and lice as well as elimination of the worms by administering an efficient anthelmintic. If this is not done, the client may find more tapeworm segments in the stool approximately 3 weeks after treatment.

Diagnosis is by finding the tapeworm segments in the feces or around the anus (Chapter 2, Fig 1). Eggs are contained in large packets that tend to remain in the segments on fecal

flotation (Fig 14). Tapeworm infection is more commonly diagnosed when the owner sees the tapeworm segments in the feces
or on the animal.

Taenia

Taenia tapeworms are the second most common tapeworms
found in dogs and cats. *Taenia pisiformis* is probably the most
common *Taenia* found in dogs, while *Taenia taeniaeformis*
(*Hydatigera taeniaeformis*) is most commonly found in cats.

Adults vary in length, depending on the species and degree of
maturity. *Taenia* segments are more or less rectangular, as
compared to the rice-shaped segments of *Dipylidium* (Chapter
2, Fig 2). The eggs of *Taenia* are small, spherical and embryonated (Fig 15). They have a thick shell with radial striations,
and measure about 37 x 32 μ. *Echinococcus* eggs cannot be
distinguished from those of *Taenia*. This is important in areas
where *Echinococcus* is enzootic.

The life cycle of *Taenia* is indirect (Fig 16, 17). The definitive
host must ingest the uncooked tissue of the intermediate host

Figure 13. Life cycle of *Dipylidium caninum*. (Courtesy of Mobay Corporation)

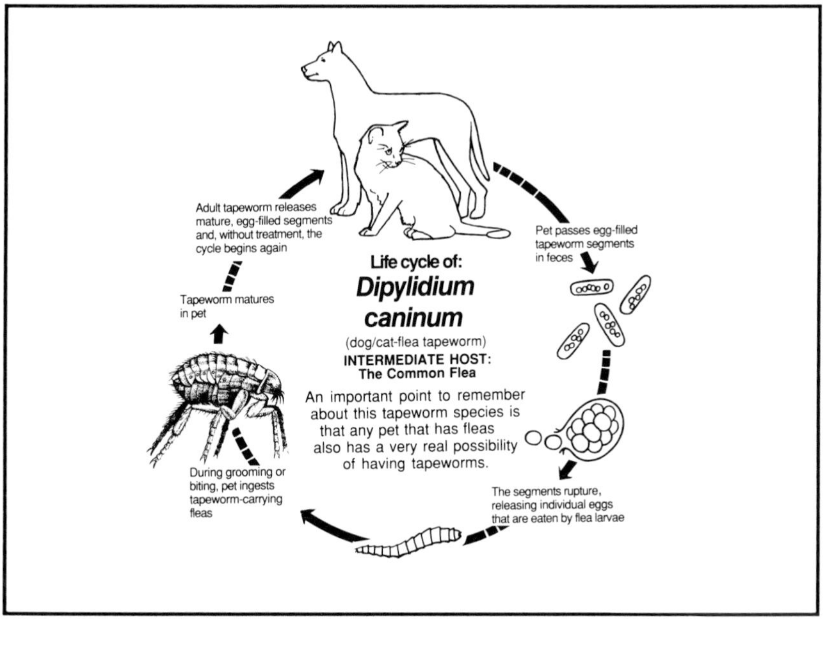

Adult tapeworm releases
mature, egg-filled segments
and, without treatment, the
cycle begins again

Tapeworm matures
in pet

During grooming or
biting, pet ingests
tapeworm-carrying
fleas

Life cycle of:
*Dipylidium
caninum*
(dog/cat-flea tapeworm)
**INTERMEDIATE HOST:
The Common Flea**
An important point to remember
about this tapeworm species is
that any pet that has fleas
also has a very real possibility
of having tapeworms.

Pet passes egg-filled
tapeworm segments
in feces

The segments rupture,
releasing individual eggs
that are eaten by flea larvae

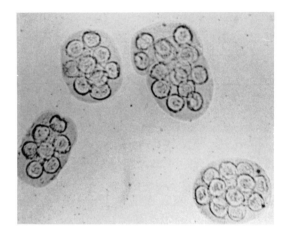

Figure 14. Packets of *Dipylidium caninum* eggs. (100X)

containing infective larvae. Maturation for most species takes about 2 months. Clinical signs in infected dogs and cats are usually minimal. Some infected dogs may "scoot" on their hindquarters as segments migrate from the rectum, but a more common cause of scooting is anal sac infection.

Echinococcus

Echinococcus granulosus and *Echinococcus multilocularis* are very small tapeworms of 5 or less segments. Only the last segment is gravid (contains eggs). *Echinococcus granulosus*

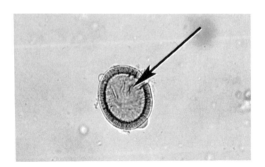

Figure 15. Egg of *Taenia*. The arrow points to the hooks (3 pairs) within the egg. (350X)

Figure 16. Life cycle of *Taenia pisiformis*. (Courtesy of Mobay Corporation)

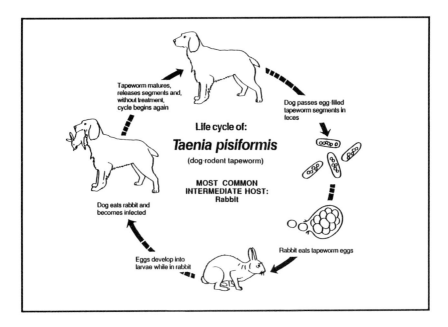

Figure 17. Life cycle of *Taenia taeniaeformis*. (Courtesy of Mobay Corporation)

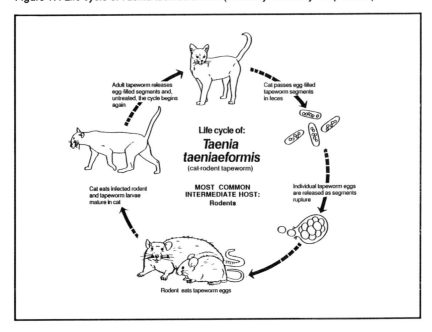

produces larvae called hydatid cysts in the intermediate hosts (cattle, sheep and occasionally people) (Fig 18). *Echinococcus multilocularis* produces alveolar hydatids in field mice, voles, lemmings, cattle, horses, swine, sheep and people (Fig 19). These tapeworms are noted for their zoonotic potential to produce hydatid cysts in people.

Because *Echinococcus* and *Taenia* eggs are so similar, eggs recovered from the feces are not diagnostic. Adult tapeworms must be collected for definitive identification. One collection method involves administration of a purgative, arecoline hydrobromide. Immunodiagnostic tests are commonly used in human medicine.

The drug of choice for treatment of tapeworm infections is praziquantel, which is 100% effective against *Taenia, Dipylidium, Mesocestoides* and *Echinococcus*. The drug kills adult *Echinococcus,* but eggs still pass in the feces for several days thereafter, so good hygiene should be practiced.

Figure 18. Life cycle of *Echinococcus granulosus*. (Courtesy of Mobay Corporation)

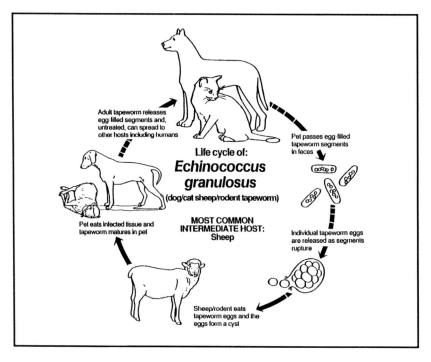

Figure 19. Life cycle of *Echinococcus multilocularis*. (Courtesy of Mobay Corporation)

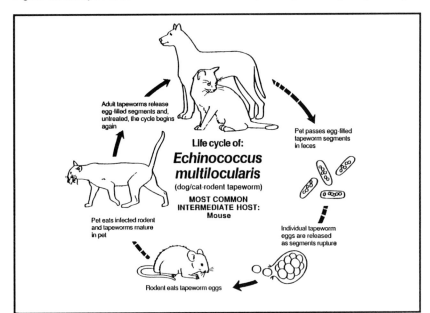

Adult tapeworms release
egg-filled segments and,
untreated, the cycle begins
again

Life cycle of:

Echinococcus multilocularis
(dog/cat-rodent tapeworm)

**MOST COMMON
INTERMEDIATE HOST:**
Mouse

Pet passes egg-filled
tapeworm segments
in feces

Individual tapeworm
eggs are released
as segments rupture

Pet eats infected rodent
and tapeworms mature
in pet

Rodent eats tapeworm eggs

Mesocestoides

Mesocestoides tapeworms are parasites of dogs, birds and occasionally people. The life cycle is not completely known, but 2 intermediate hosts appear necessary to complete it. The first intermediate host, the oribatid mite, is ingested by the second intermediate host, possibly a bird, reptile, amphibian or mammal. Cats and dogs can be intermediate hosts in this life cycle also. A larval stage, called a tetrathyridium, forms in the peritoneal cavity of mammals and reptiles, and in the air sacs of birds. The adults of *Mesocestoides corti* are capable of asexual reproduction.

Infection by adult worms in dogs is asymptomatic, while infection in people causes severe diarrhea. Severe peritonitis and ascites is common in dogs and cats infected with larvae.

Diphyllobothrium latum

Diphyllobothrium latum, the broad fish tapeworm, occurs in the small intestine of people, dogs, cats, pigs and other fish-eating mammals worldwide, but especially in the Great Lakes area of North America. The eggs in the feces are operculate and unembryonated, and measure 67-71 x 40-51 μ.

The life cycle is indirect. The unsegmented eggs take several weeks to form a coracidium similar to the miracidium of flukes. The eggs are similar but smaller than fluke eggs. The first larval stage develops in a copepod, which is ingested by the second intermediate host, a fish. A suitable definitive host, such as a dog, ingests the raw fish, and adult worms mature in 3-4 weeks. The adult worm is nonpathogenic in definitive hosts, except in people.

In people, infection occurs by ingestion of raw or undercooked fish or caviar. In people, the adult worm uses vitamin B_{12} and may cause vitamin B_{12} deficiency anemia (pernicious anemia). Diagnosis is by finding the eggs in the feces. Prevention involves freezing or thorough cooking of fish, and not feeding raw fish to animals.

Spirometra mansonoides

Spirometra tapeworms resemble *Diphyllobothrium*. The adults are similar but smaller, and the eggs have pointed ends instead of rounded ends, as with *Diphyllobothrium* (Fig 20). Adults parasitize wild carnivores, dogs and cats. The species found in raccoons, dogs and cats of North America is *Spirometra mansonoides*.

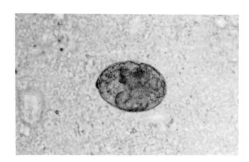

Figure 20. Egg of *Spirometra mansonoides*. (350X)

An egg passed in the feces produces a coracidium, which enters the first intermediate host, a water crustacean. The second intermediate host, usually a water snake or amphibian, develops plerocercoids that become adult worms after the intermediate host is ingested by the definitive host. The definitive host (dogs, cats, people) can be intermediate hosts as well as definitive hosts. Adult parasites are rarely pathogenic, and the plerocercoids are of public health importance. In people, migrating larvae cause a condition called sparganosis.

Hymenolepis

Hymenolepis diminuta, the rat tapeworm, is found in rats and mice. Dogs and people can become infected if they ingest the cysticercoids found in beetles, fleas or other insects. The characteristic eggs of *Hymenolepis diminuta* can be found in the feces. See Chapter 9 for more information regarding tapeworms in rodents.

Flukes

Paragonimus kellicotti

Paragonimus kellicotti is the lung fluke of dogs and cats. The primary host is probably the mink. The worms are mainly found in pairs in cysts in the lungs or susceptible hosts. Adult flukes are about 14 mm long. The eggs are golden brown and oval, with an operculum at one end, and measure 75-118 x 42-67μ (Fig 21).

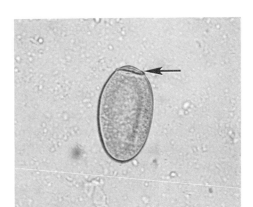

Figure 21. Egg of *Paragonimus kellicotti*. (350X)

The life cycle is indirect, with snails acting as the first inter-mediate host and crayfish as the second. Eggs pass through the cyst wall in the host's lungs and are coughed up, swallowed and passed in the feces. After a minimum of 2 weeks, the miracidium escapes and penetrates the first intermediate host, a snail. Sporocysts, rediae and cercariae develop in 11 weeks. The cer-cariae escape from the snail and penetrate into crayfish. Meta-cercariae develop in the crayfish. Suitable hosts become infected by ingesting the crayfish containing metacercariae, or drinking water containing free-swimming metacercariae. The young flukes penetrate through the intestinal wall into the peritoneal cavity, and then through the diaphragm into the lungs. Eggs are passed in the feces one month after ingestion of metacercariae.

Lung fluke infection is diagnosed by finding eggs in the sputum or feces (Fig 21). Clinical signs include lethargy and an intermittent cough. Radiographs usually reveal the cysts in the right caudal lobe of the lung. Fenbendazole is the treatment of choice, though a large dose of praziquantel also appears to be effective.

Alaria

Alaria species are flukes found in the intestinal tract of dogs, cats, foxes and mink. Wild carnivores are the usual definitive host. The adult flukes measure 2-6 mm long. The eggs are yellowish-brown, have one operculum and measure 98-134 x 62-68 μ.

Female adults produce eggs that are passed in the feces and develop into a miracidium. This penetrates into the first inter-mediate host, a snail, where it becomes a cercaria. The cercaria penetrates into the second intermediate host, usually a frog, and forms a mesocercaria. When the second intermediate host or a paratenic host containing the mesocercaria is ingested by a suitable definitive host, the mesocercaria migrates through the peritoneal cavity and lungs, and finally becomes an adult fluke in the small intestine 10 days later.

Diagnosis is made by finding the fluke eggs in the feces. Most infections are nonpathogenic. People can act as a paratenic host, with mesocercariae found in the peritoneal cavity and organs of the body.

Nanophyetus

The fluke, *Nanophyetus salmincola* (*Troglotrema salmincola*), occurs in the small intestine of dogs, cats, foxes, coyotes, raccoons, opossum, otters and minks of the Pacific Northwest. The raccoon and spotted skunk are the primary definitive hosts. The yellowish-brown eggs measure 52-82 x 32-56 μ, with an operculum at the pole.

Eggs are passed in the feces and take 3 months to develop. The first intermediate hosts are snails. Cercariae liberated from the snails swim free in the water. These cercariae penetrate the second intermediate host, a salmon. Dogs eating uncooked salmon containing metacercariae develop adult flukes in about one week.

Damage from the flukes themselves in dogs is minimal. More important, *Nanophyetus* flukes transmit the rickettsial agents of "salmon poisoning" and "Elokomin fluke fever." Salmon poisoning caused by *Neorickettsia helminthoeca* affects only canids, such as dogs, foxes and coyotes. Signs of salmon poisoning in dogs include purulent ocular discharge, vomiting, hemorrhagic diarrhea, fever and death in over 50% of affected animals. Elokomin fluke fever is similar to salmon poisoning, but has lower mortality in dogs and affects a wider range of hosts, including bears, raccoons and people.

Nanophyetus fluke infection is diagnosed by identifying the eggs in the feces. Salmon poisoning is diagnosed by finding the rickettsiae in fluid aspirated from the mandibular lymph nodes. Prevention involves not eating raw or undercooked fish.

Dicrocoelium

The lancet liver fluke, *Dicrocoelium dendriticum*, occurs in the bile duct of ruminants, pigs, deer, dogs, rabbits and occasionally people. Laboratory animals are also susceptible, and the hamster is the most satisfactory laboratory host. The distribution is worldwide, but prevalence in certain areas may be sporadic. The adult fluke is about 10 mm long. The eggs are operculated and embryonated, and measure 36-45 x 20-30 μ (Fig 22).

The life cycle is indirect. The 2 intermediate hosts required are a snail, and then an ant. Ants containing the metacercariae are ingested by a suitable host. The metacercariae are released and migrate up the bile duct to mature in 47-54 days. Most cases are asymptomatic, but edema, anemia and emaciation develop in severe cases.

Fasciola hepatica

Fasciola hepatica is the liver fluke of ruminants. The operculate eggs can be found as spurious eggs in dog and cat feces (Fig 23).

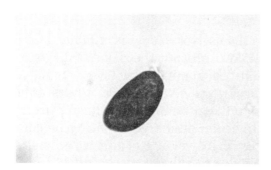

Figure 22. Egg of *Dicrocoelium dendriticum*. (350X)

Figure 23. Egg of *Fasciola hepatica*. (350X)

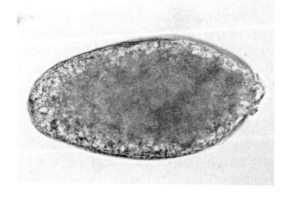

Protozoal Parasites

Isospora

Isospora is one of the protozoan parasites that can affect dogs and cats. Infections caused by *Isospora* are called coccidiosis. Transmission is by ingestion of feces or an infected prey animal. Once inside the host, *Isospora* completes its life cycle in 3-11 days.

In fresh feces, *Isospora* oocysts appear as undivided spheres (Fig 24), but older feces may contain sporulated oocysts (Fig 25). Depending on the species, *Isospora* oocysts are 10-20 μ long.

The nature of the clinical condition caused by *Isospora* is controversial. Though *Isospora* oocysts are associated with diarrhea in puppies and kittens, attempts to reproduce the disease

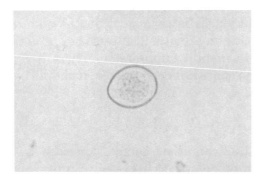

Figure 24. An *Isospora* oocyst from fresh canine feces. (350X)

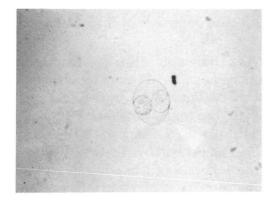

Figure 25. Sporulated *Isospora canis* oocyst. (400X)

in laboratory studies have usually failed. It is most likely, however, that *Isospora* acts, at least in part, to cause diarrhea in puppies and kittens. Other factors, such as nutrition, immune status and concurrent infection, are contributory.

Though *Isospora* infections are considered self-limiting, sulfonamides are effective in eliminating infection. Controlling the spread of *Isospora* is difficult, as it is a condition associated with kennels and veterinary hospitals. Proper hygiene in cages and pens, and disinfection with ammonium hydroxide are required.

Cryptosporidium

Cryptosporidium is another protozoan affecting small animals. Diagnosis is difficult and requires identification of very small $(5\,\mu)$, indistinct oocysts in the feces.

Signs of infection include protracted diarrhea in an otherwise healthy animal. Cryptosporidiosis is seen in neonates and is associated with immunologic immaturity. It can also be encountered in adult animals with immunosuppression. There is no effective treatment. Though is has not been proven, it should be considered a zoonotic disease.

Giardia

Giardia is a protozoan that can affect people, domestic animals and many birds. The protozoan lives in the small intestine. Infection results in a disease that may be inapparent or may result in chronic enteritis. Chronic diarrhea is a common sign of giardiasis. Transmission is by ingestion of food and water contaminated with infective feces.

Diagnosis is by observing the motile flagellate binucleate trophozoite stage in a direct saline smear of fresh diarrheic feces or by finding the cyst stage containing 2-4 nuclei on a zinc sulfate fecal flotation (Fig 26). The trophozoites are 9-21 μ long and 5-15 μ wide. Cysts measure up to 12 μ long and 8-10 μ wide. Dried saline smears can be stained with Wright's or Giemsa stain to confirm the diagnosis. Because these protozoa may be excreted intermittently, diagnosis based on observation of tro-

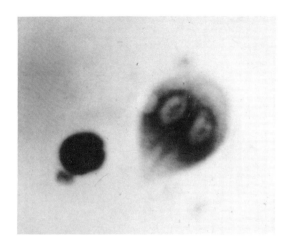

Figure 26. A *Giardia* trophozoite. (Iron hematoxylin stain, 1400X)

phozoites or cysts may be difficult. *Giardia* may be transmitted from dogs to people.

References

1. Soulsby: *Helminths, Arthropods and Protozoa of Domestic Animals.* 7th ed. Lea & Febiger, Philadelphia, 1982.

2. Georgi: Parasites of the respiratory tract. *Vet Clin No Am* 17:1421-1428, 1990.

3. Georgi: *Parasitology for Veterinarians.* 5th ed. Saunders, Philadelphia, 1985.

4. Wade and Gaafar, in Pratt: *Laboratory Procedures for Animal Health Technicians.* American Veterinary Publications, Goleta, CA, 1985.

Recommended Reading

Georgi: *Parasitology for Veterinarians.* 5th ed. Saunders, Philadelphia, 1990.

Melvin and Brooke: *Laboratory Procedures for the Diagnosis of Intestinal Parasites.* US Dept Hlth & Human Services (DHEW #76-8282), 1975.

Sloss and Kemp: *Veterinary Clinical Parasitology.* 5th ed. Iowa State Univ Press, Ames, 1978.

Soulsby: *Helminths, Arthropods and Protozoa of Domestic Animals.* 7th ed. Lea & Febiger, Philadelphia, 1982.

4

External Parasites of Dogs and Cats

L.P. Schmeitzel and P.J. Ihrke

Fleas

Fleas are blood-sucking ectoparasites of dogs, cats, birds, rabbits, rodents and people. They are vectors of several diseases, including bubonic plague. Dog and cat fleas (*Ctenocephalides canis, C felis*) are intermediate hosts of the tapeworm *Dipylidium caninum*.[2,3] Heavy infestations of fleas in young animals, especially nursing kittens, can result in severe anemia and death.

Flea saliva is both locally irritating and antigenic. Hypersensitivity to flea saliva in dogs and cats results in an intensely pruritic disease called flea-allergy dermatitis.[1]

Fleas are small, brown, wingless insects with bodies that are flattened laterally. The thorax is divided into 3 sections, each with a pair of legs. Females are larger than males.

Fleas show little host specificity and attack any source of blood if the preferred host is not available. *Ctenocephalides felis* (cat flea) and *C canis* (dog flea) both infest cats and dogs (Fig 1). By far the most common flea found on cats and dogs is *C felis*. Both species of fleas move rapidly from one area on the host to another. During physical examination, they are most easily located on the rump and ventral abdomen.

Sticktight fleas (*Echidnophaga gallinacea*) are found on birds and may attack cats and dogs (Fig 2). The female attaches to the skin and does not move rapidly to other areas.[3]

Pulex irritans (human flea) occasionally attacks cats and dogs.

Specific identification of different species of fleas requires the expertise of an entomologist.[2] However, this is rarely necessary clinically.

To collect adult fleas, spray the haircoat with an insecticide and, in a few minutes, dead fleas will drop from the host.

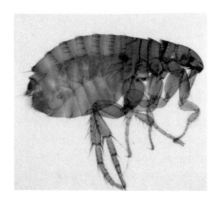

Figure 1. *Ctenocephalides felis* (cat flea). (Courtesy of R. Bell, Texas A&M Univ)

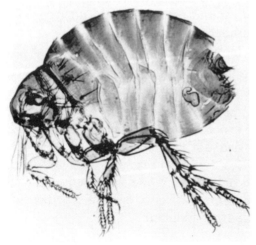

Figure 2. *Echidnophaga gallinacea* (sticktight flea). (Courtesy of R. Bell, Texas A&M Univ)

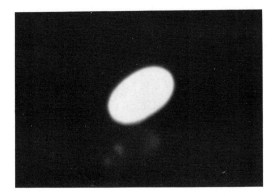

Figure 3. Flea eggs are ovoid, white and glistening. (Courtesy of L. Dunning, Univ California)

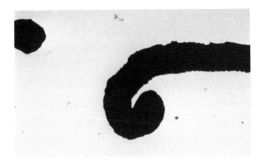

Figure 4. Flea droppings appear as reddish-black, comma-shaped casts.

Flea eggs are rarely found on the host because they do not have a sticky coating. The eggs are ovoid, white and glistening (Fig 3).

Fecal droppings (flea dirt) from adult female fleas consist of reddish-black, comma-shaped casts of dehydrated blood (Fig 4).[1] These fecal casts are found in the haircoat of cats and dogs infested with fleas. When this material is placed on white paper or a slide with a drop of water, the water turns reddish brown as the feces dissolve.

This procedure is an excellent aid to help convince owners that their pet is infested with fleas.

Ticks

Ticks are blood-sucking arthropod ectoparasites. Most ticks are not host specific. Ticks transmit many bacterial, viral, rickettsial and protozoal diseases. Heavy infestation may result in severe anemia.[3] Tick paralysis, an ascending flaccid paralysis, is caused by a neurotoxin in the saliva of 12 different ixodid species (hard ticks). Recovery is rapid after the ticks are removed.

All ticks have a 4-stage life cycle; the egg, the 6-legged larva (seed tick), the 8-legged nymph, and the 8-legged adult. Ticks are identified as 1-host, 2-host or 3-host ticks, depending upon the number of different hosts required to complete their life cycle.

There are 2 main families of parasitic ticks: Ixodidae (hard ticks) and Argasidae (soft ticks). Ixodid ticks (hard ticks) have a hard scutum or chitinous shield that covers a small area behind the head of females and immature stages, and covers the entire dorsum of males. Most hard ticks require 3 different hosts to complete their life cycle.[1] The larva, nymph and adult feed only once during each stage.[4]

There are 13 species of economically important ticks in the Ixodidae family, including *Rhipicephalus sanguineus, Ixodes scapularis, Dermacentor* spp and *Amblyomma* spp. Most of these ticks gain access to the host outdoors, except for *R sanguineus*, which can infest buildings.

Rhipicephalus sanguineus, the brown dog tick, is widely distributed in North America. This tick can survive outdoors and may be a serious problem in kennels and households. Though *R sanguineus* is a 3-host tick, all 3 stages primarily parasitize the dog, as well as cats, horses, rabbits and people. The tick has a vase-shaped base of the capitulum (head) and has no white markings on the dorsal shield (inornate scutum) (Fig 5). The major importance of differentiating *R sanguineus* from other ixodids is that this tick can result in severe kennel infestations.[3]

Dermacentor variabilis, the American dog tick, is also widely distributed in North America, and is especially common on the Atlantic coast. These ticks, unlike *R sanguineus*, only inhabit shrubs and grasses.[1,2] The adult tick primarily parasitizes dogs but also infests wild mammals, cattle, horses and people. The immature stages primarily parasitize field mice. *Dermacentor* spp have a rectangular base of the capitulum and white markings on the dorsal shield (ornate scutum) (Fig 6).[1,4] *Dermacentor variabilis* is rarely an environmental problem. If large numbers of *D variabilis* are found on an animal, an outside area, such as a field, is the most likely source of the ticks.

Figure 5. *Rhipicephalus sanguineus* has no white markings on its inornate dorsal shield. Male on left and female on right. (Courtesy of L. Dunning, Univ California)

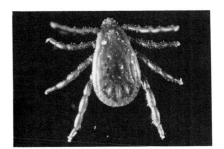
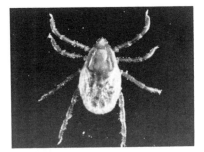

Figure 6. *Dermacentor variabilis* has white markings on its ornate dorsal shield. Male on left and female on right. (Courtesy of L. Dunning, Univ California)

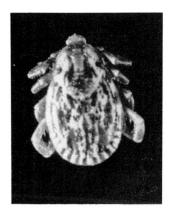
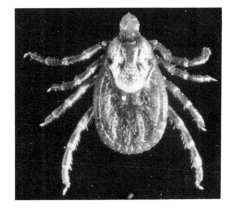

Before collection, hard ticks should be sprayed with an insecticide or soaked with alcohol. The head is grasped with forceps and gentle traction is applied.

Argasid ticks (soft ticks) lack a dorsal scutum, and have a leathery consistency and ventral capitulum. Only one species, *Otobius megnini*, the spinose ear tick, is of veterinary importance (Fig 7). It is most prevalent in the southwestern United States. Only larval and nymphal stages are found in the external ear canal of dogs, cats, cattle and horses. The immature stages may feed repeatedly, but adults do not feed.[1,4]

The spinose ear tick causes severe irritation to the external ear canal. Neurologic signs, including paralysis and convulsions, have been reported in several species infested with spinose ear ticks.[1] Blunt instruments should be used to remove these ticks from the ear canal. Care should be taken to prevent damaging the tympanic membrane during extraction.

Lice

Lice are not common parasites in the United States. They spend their entire life cycle on the host. Females attach their eggs (nits) to the hairs or feathers of the host. Immature forms undergo several molts, with minor morphologic changes, before

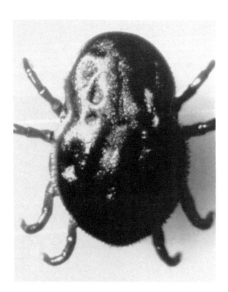

Figure 7. *Otobius megnini* nymph. This tick has a leathery consistency. (Courtesy of Extension Vet Med, Univ California)

becoming adults. Lice are very host specific, which aids species identification.[2,4]

Lice are dorsoventrally flattened, wingless insects. Their bodies are divided into a head, thorax and abdomen, with 3 pairs of legs attached to the thorax. The length of adults varies from 1 to 5 mm, depending on the species.

There are 2 suborders of lice: Anoplura (sucking lice) and Mallophaga (biting lice). Anoplura or sucking lice are larger than biting lice. They have elongated heads, with piercing mouthparts, and pincer-like claws adapted for clinging to the host's hairs (Fig 8).[4] These lice are gray to red, depending on the amount of blood they have ingested.[2] Various species of sucking lice infest all species of domestic animals, except birds and cats. Sucking lice move slowly from one area to another on the host.

Mallophaga or biting lice are usually yellow and have a large, rounded head, with mandible-like mouthparts adapted for chewing and biting (Fig 9). Several species have legs adapted for clasping, while others have legs adapted for moving rapidly.[4] Biting lice are found on cattle, sheep, goats, horses, dogs, cats and birds.

Figure 8. The sucking louse of cattle, *Linognathus vituli*. Note the piercing mouthparts and pincer-like claws. (Courtesy of Extension Vet Med, Univ California)

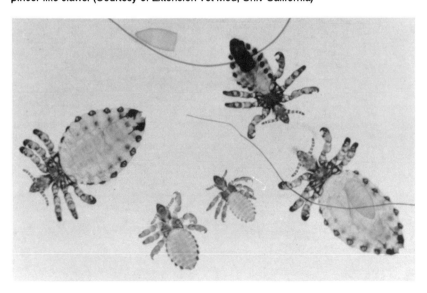

Specific genus and species identification of each louse is difficult and is not as important clinically as differentiating the biting species from the more pathogenic sucking species.[1,2,4] Dogs are infested by one common biting louse, *Trichodectes canis,* and one common sucking louse, *Linognathus setosus.* Cats usually are infested only by the biting louse, *Felicola subrostratus* (Fig 9).[1]

Adult lice may be seen with the unaided eye with some difficulty. The small, white eggs (nits) may be seen attached to the hairs or feathers. A hand lens and good lighting facilitate detection of lice or nits (Fig 10).

The lice and eggs attached to the hairs may be collected with forceps and placed on a slide with mineral oil. The slide is examined at low magnification (4X-10X objectives) (Fig 10).

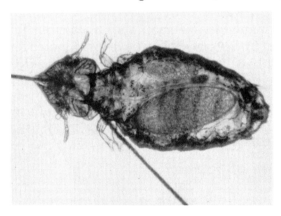

Figure 9. The biting louse of cats, *Felicola subrostratus.* Note the large, rounded head and the mandible-like mouthparts. An egg is also shown. (Courtesy of R. Bell, Texas A&M Univ)

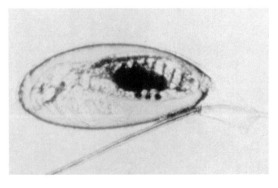

Figure 10. A louse egg (nit) attached to a hair. (Courtesy of R. Bell, Texas A&M Univ)

Mites

Demodex

Demodex mites parasitize people and most domestic animals. In many species they are considered nonpathogenic in small numbers and a part of the normal cutaneous fauna. These mites are host specific and are not transmissible. The clinical disease, caused by an increased number of mites, is called demodicosis.[1,4] *Demodex* spp are elongated, with short, stubby legs (Fig 11). Adults and nymphs have 8 legs, and larvae have 6 legs. The adults are about $250\,\mu$ long. The eggs are fusiform (Fig 12). Dogs are commonly affected by *D canis*. The mites may be found in small numbers on normal skin in dogs. However, the presence of 1-2 mites in a series of 10 scrapings from abnormal skin does not indicate that demodicosis is present.

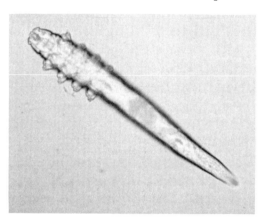

Figure 11. *Demodex* mites are elongated and have short, stubby legs.

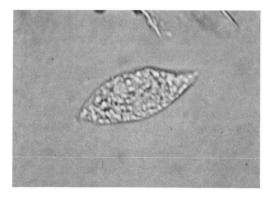

Figure 12. *Demodex* eggs are fusiform.

Demodex lives in hair follicles and sebaceous glands. There are 2 forms in dogs: localized and generalized. The main clinical signs of localized demodicosis are patchy alopecia. Generalized demodicosis is characterized by diffuse alopecia, erythema and secondary bacterial infection. An inherited defect in the animal's immune system is believed to be an important factor in the pathogenesis of generalized demodicosis.[1]

Areas of skin with altered pigmentation, obstructed hair follicles, erythema or alopecia should be scraped. In localized demodicosis, the areas most commonly affected are the forelegs and perioral and periorbital regions. In generalized demodicosis, the entire body may be affected, however; the feet and face usually are most severely involved. Apparently normal skin should also be scraped to ascertain if the disease is generalized. The areas should be clipped and a fold of skin gently squeezed to express any mites from the hair follicles. The scraping is done as previously described (see Chapter 2). Scrapings should be continued until capillary blood oozing is evident, as demodectic mites live deep in the hair follicles.[1]

The mites on the slide should be counted and a live:dead ratio calculated. The presence of any immature stages or eggs should also be noted. A decrease in the number of eggs and live mites during therapy is a good prognostic sign.

Cats are affected by 2 species of demodectic mites: *Demodex cati* and an unnamed *Demodex* species. *Demodex cati* is an elongated mite similar to *D canis*. The new *Demodex* species isolated from cats has a broad, blunted abdomen as compared to the elongated abdomen of *Demodex cati*.[5] Demodicosis caused by either species is rare in cats. In the localized form, there are patchy areas of alopecia, erythema and occasionally crusting on the head, ears and neck. In the generalized form, the alopecia, erythema and crusting may involve the entire body. Demodicosis may also cause ceruminous otitis externa in cats.[6]

Sarcoptes and *Notoedres*

The family Sarcoptidae includes the genera *Sarcoptes* and *Notoedres*. These mites are relatively host specific and spread by direct contact. The mites burrow within the epidermis. The entire 5-stage life cycle is spent on the host and includes the egg, a 6-legged larva, 2 8-legged nymphal stages, and an 8-legged adult. Development from egg to adult takes about 17 days.[3]

The disease caused by *Sarcoptes scabiei* is called scabies, sarcoptic acariasis or sarcoptic mange (Fig 13). It is an intensely pruritic disease. The mites are often difficult to demonstrate on multiple skin scrapings. For this reason, scabies is often tentatively diagnosed by the lesions and their distribution.[4] Because scabies mites can be found only about 50% of the time, irrespective of the number of scrapings, dogs with suspected scabies should be treated on the basis of clinical signs.

All mites in this family may occasionally be transmitted to other species, including people.[1,7] Scabies is one of the most common transmissible pruritic canine skin diseases. It generally affects all dogs in a household and is one of the 2 most common small animal zoonoses. Carrier states may exist.

Canine scabies is caused by *Sarcoptes scabiei* var *canis*. The lesions consist of an erythematous, papular rash. Scaling, crusting and self-trauma are common. Though the entire body may be affected, the ears, lateral elbows and ventral abdomen are recommended scraping sites, as they are more likely to harbor mites than other areas.[1] Occasionally the owners are affected by the mites, but the disease is considered self-limiting in people.[1] Cats are not thought to be affected by *Sarcoptes scabiei* var *canis*.

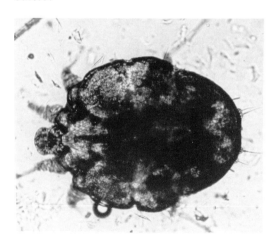

Figure 13. *Sarcoptes scabiei* var *canis*. These mites are oval and have long, unsegmented pedicles, with suckers on several pairs of legs. The anus is terminal.

Feline scabies (notoedric mange) is an uncommon skin disease with enzootic foci in various areas of the United States. The causative mite, *Notoedres cati*, affects the head and forelegs (Fig 14).

Areas with an erythematous, papular rash and crusts should be scraped. Multiple skin scrapings are needed to demonstrate sarcoptic mites. Notoedric mites are easier to demonstrate than sarcoptic mites in dogs. Adult sarcoptic mites are oval and about 200-400 μ in diameter, with 4 pairs of legs (Fig 15). Females have long, unsegmented pedicles, with suckers on 2 pairs of legs. Males have long, unsegmented pedicles, with suckers on 3 pairs of legs. The anus is located on the caudal end of the body.[2]

Adult notoedric mites are similar to sarcoptic mites but are smaller, and the anus is located dorsad (Fig 14). The 8-legged

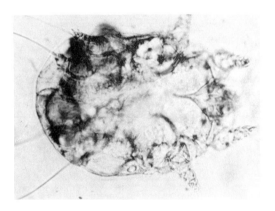

Figure 14. *Notoedres cati* mites also have long, unsegmented pedicles, with suckers on several pairs of legs. The anus is dorsal; *Sarcoptes scabiei* has a terminal anus. (Courtesy of R. Bell, Texas A&M Univ)

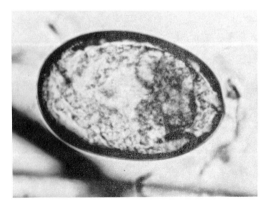

Figure 15. Eggs from sarcoptic mites are oval. This is a *Notoedres cati* egg. (Courtesy of R. Bell, Texas A&M Univ)

nymphs of both sarcoptic and notoedric mites are smaller than the adults. The 6-legged larva lacks a caudal pair of legs. The eggs of both sarcoptic and notoedric mites are oval (Fig 15).[1,4]

Otodectes

The family Psoroptidae includes the genus *Otodectes*. These mites have 5 developmental stages, including the egg, a 6-legged larva, 2 8-legged nymphal stages, and an 8-legged adult.[2,3] Otodectic mites live in the external ear canal.

Otodectes cynotis, the ear mite, is a common cause of otitis externa in cats and dogs. Though they are found primarily in the external ear canal, rarely they may be found on other parts of the body.[1,3] These mites are not host specific and are readily transmitted between cats and dogs.[1]

Otodectic mites cause intense irritation and thick, dry, black crusts in the ear canals. Through an otoscope, the mites appear as white, mobile objects.

To collect ear mites, a cotton-tipped applicator is moistened with mineral oil, introduced into the external ear canal and gently rotated. The material obtained is then spread on a microscope slide with additional mineral oil. A glass coverslip is applied and the material is examined at low power (10X objective). Otodectic mites are about 450 μ long (Fig 16). Females have short, unsegmented pedicles, with suckers on 2 of their 4

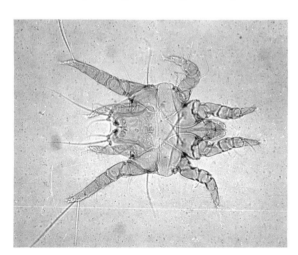

Figure 16. *Otodectes cynotis* male. (Courtesy of M.M.J. Laviopierre, Univ California)

pairs of legs. The fourth pair of legs is rudimentary. Males have short, unsegmented pedicles, with suckers on all 4 pairs of legs.[2]

Cheyletiella

Cheyletiella spp (walking dandruff mite) are contagious mites that live on the skin surface. These mites are relatively host specific and cause excessive scaling and crusting on the dorsal aspects of the body, with a variable degree of pruritus.[1]

The most common species in dogs is *Cheyletiella yasguri*, in cats is *C blakei* and in rabbits is *C parasitovorax*.[1,2] The mites may be seen with the aid of a hand magnifier. Alternatively, superficial skin scrapings or cellophane-tape preparations may be examined microscopically (see Chapter 2).[1]

Cheyletiella spp have longer legs and are larger (about 450 μ long) than *Sarcoptes scabiei* (Fig 17). The horn-like accessory mouthparts make these mites very distinctive.[1,2,4]

Trombicula

Only the larvae of trombiculid mites (chiggers) are parasitic on animals and people. The nymphs and adults are free living. The larvae are most common in the late summer and early fall,

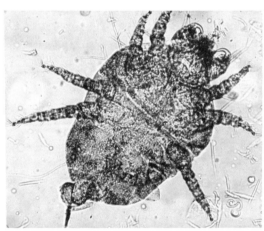

Figure 17. *Cheyletiella parasitovorax*, the walking dandruff mite.

and are transmitted by direct contact with foliage in fields and heavy underbrush.

The most common trombiculid mite affecting animals and people is *Trombicula alfreddugesi* (North American chigger). Lesions consist of an erythematous, often pruritic papular rash on the ventrum, face, feet and legs.[1] The orange-red larvae may also be found in the ears of cats.

The larvae remain attached to the skin only for several hours.[2] Consequently, the disease may be difficult to diagnose, as the pruritus persists after the larvae have fallen off. However, scraping an orange dot on the skin may yield a 6-legged larva.[1] Trombiculid larvae are about 450 μ long and vary in color from yellowish to red (Fig 18).

Miscellaneous External Parasites

Pelodera

Pelodera strongyloides (*Rhabditis strongyloides*) is a free-living saprophytic nematode. Adults live in moist organic debris, such as straw. Larvae invade the skin of dogs housed on this type of bedding. *Pelodera* dermatitis (rhabditic dermatitis) is rare and primarily seen in the Midwest. The lesions consist of a pruritic, erythematous, papular rash over the ventral contact areas.

Multiple skin scrapings of affected areas are required to demonstrate the small larvae.[1] Larvae of *P strongyloides* are

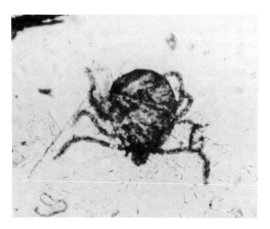

Figure 18. *Trombicula* (chigger) larva.

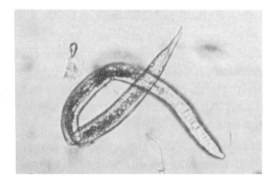

Figure 19. *Pelodera strongyloides* larva. (Courtesy of J. MacDonald, Auburn Univ)

about 596-600 μ long (Fig 19).[5] They must be differentiated from microfilariae of *Dirofilaria immitis* (heartworm) and *Dipetalonema reconditum*, which may also be rarely found on a skin scraping (see Chapter 2).

Cuterebra

Larvae of *Cuterebra* flies infest rabbits, squirrels, mice, cats and occasionally dogs.[4] They are 2-3 cm long, with large, black spines.[4] Eggs are laid by adults in the soil of rodent burrows. Larvae penetrate the host's skin and live in a subcutaneous pseudocyst, with a fistula communicating with the outside. Pets contract this disease while investigating rodent burrows. The most commonly affected site is the subcutaneous tissue of the neck. Most cases occur during the summer.[1]

Larvae are often discovered during physical examination and are removed surgically. The fistula is enlarged and the larva is removed with forceps.

References

1. Muller *et al: Small Animal Dermatology.* 4th ed. Saunders, Philadelphia, 1989.

2. Sloss and Kemp: *Veterinary Clinical Parasitology.* 5th ed. Iowa State Univ Press, Ames, 1978.

3. Soulsby: *Helminths, Arthropods and Protozoa of Domestic Animals.* 7th ed. Lea & Febiger, Philadelphia, 1982.

4. Georgi: *Parasitology for Veterinarians.* 4th ed. Saunders, Philadelphia, 1985.

5. *JAAHA* 18:405, 1982.

6. *JAAHA* 16:367, 1980.

7. Blood *et al: Veterinary Medicine.* 6th ed. Bailliere Tindall, London, 1983.

5

Internal Parasites of Horses

T.R. Bello

Horses may be infected by a variety of internal parasites. The most common are intestinal threadworms (*Strongyloides westeri*), ascarids (*Parascaris equorum*), bots (*Gasterophilus* spp), pinworms (*Oxyuris equi* and *Probstmayria vivipara*), stomach worms (*Habronema* spp and *Trichostrongylus axei*), tapeworms (*Anoplocephala* spp), and the small and large strongyles.

Parasites cause a variety of host reactions, ranging from no apparent ill effect to severe tissue destruction and death. The extent of injury is related to the pathogenic potential of the individual parasite species as well as the number of parasites involved in the infection. Severity of infection is also related to the age and acquired or natural resistance status of the horse, and the duration over which the infection is obtained. Injurious effects, such as blood loss, tissue destruction, mechanical obstruction, intoxication and competitive uptake of food, are commonly attributed to the adult or mature stages of parasites. However, the greatest damage may be done by larval stages rather than by adult parasites.

Infection usually is diagnosed by microscopic examination of slides prepared by concentration and flotation of parasite eggs from feces. Strongyle species may be further identified by microscopic examination of infective larvae cultured from feces, which is usually performed in research laboratories. Bot infection cannot be detected by fecal examination, but the presence of botfly eggs on the hairs of the horse for longer than one week is cause to presume infection.

Large Strongyles[1]

The large strongyle group is comprised of only 3 species. Two of these, *Strongylus vulgaris* and *S edentatus,* are quite prevalent, whereas the third species, *S equinus,* has a limited distribution in the United States. Large strongyles are the most injurious of all equine parasites, primarily because of the widespread, prolonged migration of larval stages in the host's internal organs. Severe tissue damage is produced by seemingly small numbers of larvae. Adult large strongyles become firmly attached to the mucosa of the cecum and ventral large colon, where they damage the mucosa while sucking blood.

Life Cycle: The life cycles of the large strongyles are essentially the same except the prepatent periods vary. Adult strongyles produce eggs that are passed in the feces. Under ideal conditions, infective larvae develop on pasture in one week. These larvae crawl up the blades of grass and are ingested by horses. Fourth-stage larvae migrate through the circulatory system and eventually reach the large intestine where they mature to adults.

Adult *Strongylus vulgaris* worms are the smallest of the 3 large strongyles but are the most pathogenic. Adult females of *Strongylus vulgaris* are larger than adult males, and are approximately 20-24 mm long. Adult females of *Strongylus equinus* are the largest, measuring approximately 38-47 mm in length.

Strongylus vulgaris has the shortest prepatent period of about 6 months, while *Strongylus edentatus* has the longest prepatent period of about 11 months.

Diagnosis: For practical purposes, strongyle eggs in the feces can be regarded as presumptive evidence of the presence of large strongyles because they generally are found with small strongyles. Due to the prolonged prepatent periods associated with large strongyle infections, eggs of *S vulgaris, S equinus* and *S edentatus* do not appear in foals younger than 6, 9 and 11

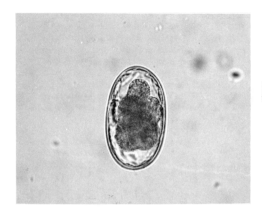

Figure 1. A strongyle egg from fresh equine feces. (350X)

months, respectively. In yearlings and older animals, large strongyle eggs ordinarily constitute less than 10% of the total number of strongyle eggs in a given fecal sample.

The eggs of *Strongylus* species are typical strongyle eggs resembling hookworm eggs of dogs (Fig 1). Strongyle eggs are elliptic, with a thin wall enclosing many cells. They are 35-55 μ wide by 70-125 μ long. The strongyle eggs of horses cannot be differentiated from each other.

Small Strongyles[1]

Horses throughout the world are parasitized by a varying mixture of small strongyles comprising 12 genera and 52 species.[2] As these parasites cannot be differentiated from each other or from large strongyles by microscopic examination of eggs, reports usually indicate numbers of "strongyle eggs." The general inference of such observations is that the environment may be contaminated with feces containing the eggs of *Strongylus vulgaris, S edentatus* and/or *S equinus*, in addition to those of small strongyles.

Life Cycle: Of the 52 species of small strongyles, just over 10 are abundant and commonly recorded.[2,3] All small strongyles have a direct life cycle. Eggs laid by adult females are passed in equine feces to develop on pasture. Hatched larvae go through 2 stages, during which they feed on bacteria and grow. Second-stage larvae develop into third-stage (infective) larvae, retaining the second-stage cuticle as an enveloping sheath. Nonfeeding infective larvae migrate up grass blades and are eaten by horses. When eaten, the larvae exsheath and become infective third-stage larvae. These invade the wall of the large colon and cecum to develop into the fourth stage. The larvae stay in the gut wall for 1-2 months, depending on the species. They emerge into the gut lumen, molt into the fifth stage and become sexually mature during a period of 5-12 weeks. Small strongyles do not suck blood and do not attach to the intestinal wall.

Ascarids[1]

Infections with large roundworms (*Parascaris equorum*) are very common in foals, sucklings, weanlings and, to a lesser extent, yearlings and 2-year-olds. Resistance to ascarid infection commonly develops by 6 months of age, with a concurrent rapid decrease in ascarid egg numbers.[4] Marked resistance to *P equorum* infection develops by 6 months, even in the absence of previous exposure to ascarids.[5] Mature horses are occasionally reinfected when they return from show circuits or the race track to the farm, where they are reexposed to ascarid eggs. The extent of infections varies widely in foals, ranging from a few worms to a few thousand. Both mature and immature worms can be present simultaneously.

Life Cycle: Mature ascarids inhabit the cranial portion of the small intestine. They are the largest parasite of the horse, and females become as long as 10-12 inches. They are very prolific egg layers, producing 200,000 eggs/female/day. Eggs are passed in the feces and, under favorable environmental conditions, embryonate and develop to the infective stage in 2 weeks. The eggs do not hatch and the infective larvae are retained in the thick egg shells. They are very resistant to adverse environments and can live for years in stables or on pastures.

The source of early infections is environmental contamination from previous crops of foals. The foals ingest the embryonated eggs in contaminated feed or water, by licking stall walls, or from the contaminated udder of the dam. The eggs hatch in the intestine, releasing larvae that penetrate the intestinal wall. They migrate though the portal veins to the liver 2 days after infection and then from the liver to the lungs 7-14 days after infection.[6] After further growth and development in the lungs, larvae return to the small intestine via the tracheoesophageal route by day 17. As the worms mature in the small intestine, their numbers decrease rapidly due to elimination. Patent ascarid infections occur in foals 10-13 weeks old.

Clinical Signs: The primary dangers of ascarid infection are acute rupture of the small intestine caused by masses of worms, with resultant peritonitis, and unthriftiness from chronic malabsorption of nutrients.

Motility of the intestine may be slowed or halted, producing death by impaction (Fig 2). Organophosphates (dichlorvos, trichlorfon) kill ascarids, resulting in rupture of the cuticle and sudden release of antigenic fluid into the intestine. If these drugs are given to a foal with a large number of ascarids in a hypomotile intestine, the resulting reaction may be fatal.

Diagnosis: Infection with mature ascarids is verified by finding the characteristic thick-shelled eggs in the feces (Fig 3).

Mature ascarids are commonly passed in feces and are readily recognized by their size. Immature stages can be confused with mature pinworms. The distinguishing feature is the more uniform body diameter and blunt tail of ascarids, which contrast with the long, tapered, sharp tail of the female pinworm.

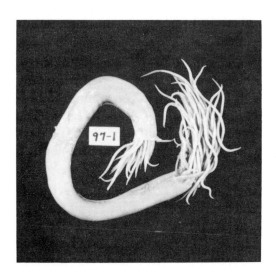

Figure 2. Impaction of the small intestine by *Parascaris equorum* in a 4-month-old foal.

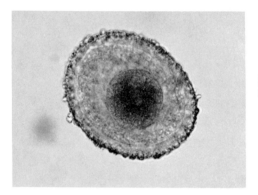

Figure 3. An egg of *Parascaris equorum*. (350X)

Pinworms[1]

Oxyuris equi

The common pinworm, *Oxyuris equi,* is an ubiquitous parasite of horses. Adult pinworms are common in foals but relatively uncommon in mature horses. Seemingly heavy infections
of larval oxyurids, numbering in excess of 20,000, occur in horses
of all ages, however.

Life Cycle: Adult pinworms live in the dorsal large and small
colon. Gravid females migrate to the rectum and anus. Because
they are quite fragile, they rupture easily, and their eggs and
other contents are deposited on the host's perineum. Some adult
worms are voided intact in the feces.

Pinworm eggs are sticky and adhere to stable walls, fixtures,
fences and bedding. Their development is rapid, requiring only
3-5 days to contain larvae. Infective eggs in contaminated bedding or water, or on walls and fences, are then ingested. The
larvae develop in the colon to the fourth stage in 3-10 days
without invading the mucosa and are sexually mature about 5
months after infection.

Clinical Signs: The principal effect of pinworm infection is
anal irritation caused by the deposits of ruptured females. The
pruritus may be intense, causing the horse to rub its rear
quarters on any available object. This results in loss of hair from
the tail, giving it the characteristic "rat-tailed" appearance.

Oxyuris infection does not otherwise cause any specific clinical signs.

Diagnosis: Oxyurid eggs are not ordinarily seen in routine fecal flotations, even in known infected animals. Use of transparent tape helps detect eggs in the perianal region (see Chapter 2). Female worms are passed spontaneously and are frequently seen in fresh feces. Their gray-white color and sharp tails are distinguishing features. Tail-rubbing and loss of hair from the tail provide presumptive evidence of pinworm infection.

Probstmayria vivipara

The minute pinworm, *Probstmayria vivipara,* is unique among nematode parasites because its entire life cycle is completed within the large intestine. Adult females produce sexually mature offspring. This explains why infections involving worms numbering in the millions are encountered but does not explain the mechanism of transmission from horse to horse, by ingestion of fresh feces.

Infections with *P vivipara* occur sporadically, but studies have been hampered because diagnosis cannot be made by fecal flotation. Finding the worms during necropsy is the only way of verifying the infection. The worms are only 2-3 mm long and are easily overlooked unless a pea-sized portion of colon contents is well diluted with water in a Petri dish and examined under a dissection microscope at 10X magnification. Pathogenic effects have not been described and *P vivipara* is believed harmless.

Bots

Virtually every horse in temperate climates, except those confined indoors, become infected with bots. May foals less than 18 hours old can have botfly eggs deposited on the hairs of the abdomen, shoulders and legs. Therefore, a 7-day-old foal can have a significant bot infection. It is unusual to perform a necropsy on a horse at any time of the year and not find bots in the stomach. Two species, *Gasterophilus intestinalis* and *G nasalis,* are prevalent throughout the United States and other parts of the world. A third species, *G haemorrhoidalis,* is less common in this country.

Life Cycle: These parasites produce one generation a year. The bots spend the winter in the stomach of horses in temperate climates. The season of botfly activity and egg deposition is prolonged in these areas, extending from late spring until late fall. The transmission season of *G intestinalis* is further extended several weeks into early winter by persistence of viable larvae in egg cases on the hair.

Embryonated eggs of *G intestinalis* do not hatch spontaneously but must be stimulated by the sudden increase in temperature, moisture and action of the lips of the horse. The eggs of *G nasalis* hatch after one week of development, when they contain infective first-stage larvae. In either case, first-stage larvae invade the gingivae and burrow through the dorsum of the tongue. After 3 weeks of growth, they emerge from the caudal aspect of the tongue as second-stage larvae and crawl down the esophagus to the stomach. Further growth and development to third-stage larvae occur in the stomach in 3-4 weeks. Third-stage larvae remain in the stomach up to 10 months before they detach from the mucosa and pass in the feces.

Second- and third-stage larvae form typical clusters. The larvae of *G intestinalis* prefer the esophageal portion of the stomach, and larvae of *G nasalis* prefer the pylorus and duodenum, just caudal to the pyloric sphincter (Fig 4). Larvae of both species produce deep pits that can perforate the wall to cause fatal peritonitis.

Diagnosis: Bot infection cannot be diagnosed by fecal flotation unless a bot happens to appear in the sample. The presence of eggs on the hair for at least one week is sufficient evidence to indicate internal infection (Fig 5).

Threadworms[1]

Strongyloides westeri

Strongyloides westeri is a common parasite in the small intestinal mucosa of young foals. Foals are usually infected by nursing the milk of an infected mare 4-47 days after foaling.[7] Additional infection may be by consumption of debris contaminated with infective larvae or by percutaneous penetration of infective

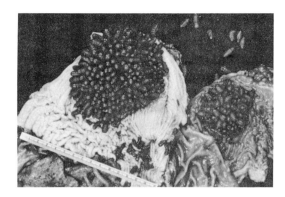

Figure 4. Clusters of bots, *Gasterophilus intestinalis*, in the stomach (left) and *Gasterophilus nasalis* in the duodenum (right).

larvae. *Strongyloides* is not transmitted in colostrum. *Strongyloides* eggs are found in feces 6-10 days after experimental infection.

Egg production peaks from weeks 3 to 6. Egg counts then rapidly decrease from weeks 7 to 16, and some foals lose the infection by week 10. The foals are thereafter resistant to reinfection. The immunity acquired from this infection is strong.[8]

Infective *Strongyloides* larvae can penetrate human skin causing cutaneous larva migrans, a possible occupational dis-

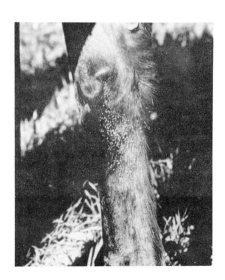

Figure 5. *Gasterophilus intestinalis* eggs on the hairs of the leg.

ease of equine practitioners, laboratory workers and stable personnel.

Diagnosis: Embryonated eggs may be observed in the feces of infected foals (Fig 6). A characteristic diagonal line formed by the folded larva aids identification.

Stomach Worms

Habronema and *Draschia*

Three species of spirurids (*Habronema muscae, Habronema majus,* and *Draschia megastoma*) are found in the equine stomach. In addition, the infective larvae of these species often invade skin wounds, causing the condition commonly referred to as "summer sores." Its seasonal prevalence is associated with the occurrence of house and stable flies that act as intermediate hosts. Larvae may invade eyes and cause persistent conjunctivitis. Pulmonary abscesses result when they invade the lungs. Parenteral invasions of larvae are considered aberrant because it is believed that only larvae gaining direct access to the stomach complete their development. In the stomach, the 2 species of *Habronema* become embedded in mucous exudate normally covering the glandular areas. *Draschia megastoma* produces abscesses in the stomach wall, where worms live in colonies.

Diagnosis: Diagnosis of stomach worm infection is difficult because their eggs are not recovered in routine fecal flotations.

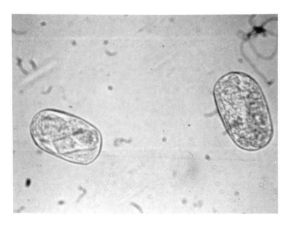

Figure 6. Eggs of the threadworm, *Strongyloides*. (400X)

When they are observed, these eggs are much longer than wide and contain a fully formed larva surrounded by a very thin shell wall (Fig 7). The larvae may also be hatched out of their eggs, even in fresh feces. Egg length is about 50 μ.

Demonstration of larvae that develop in houseflies feeding on a suspected sample may be used in diagnosis. Cutaneous infections can be diagnosed by scrapings or biopsy.

Trichostrongylus axei

The minute stomach worm, *Trichostrongylus axei,* affects cattle, sheep and goats as well as horses. Equine infections are light, even when cattle and horses graze pastures on a rotational basis. Its life cycle corresponds to that described for the small strongyles. The larvae do not migrate and the entire development occurs in about 3 weeks in the stomach.

Diagnosis: Diagnosis is by demonstration of the characteristic eggs in fecal flotations. They resemble strongyle eggs except that one side is flattened, one end is pointed, and they are more advanced in development. The eggs are all oval, thin shelled and 70-120 μ long, with contents divided into 4 or more cells (Fig 8).

Trichostrongyle larvae hatched from the eggs in fecal culture may be used for identification. The infective larvae of *T axei* have short tails, in contrast to the long whip-like tails of strongyle larvae.

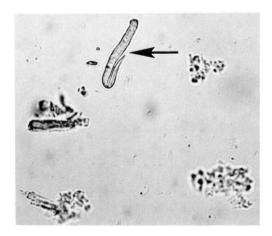

Figure 7. An egg of *Habronema* (arrow). Note the very thin shell surrounding the enclosed larva. (350X)

Tapeworms[1]

Anoplocephala

Of the 2 species of tapeworms most frequently found in the digestive tract of horses, *Anoplocephala perfoliata* occurs more frequently than *A magna* throughout the temperate zones of the world. The incidence of *A magna* may cycle every few years, whereas *A perfoliata* is found more consistently from year to year. Infections by *A perfoliata* are usually more massive than those by *A magna*. The latter is a large worm, 12 or more inches long, and is found in the caudal half of the small intestine (Fig 9). *Anoplocephala perfoliata* is only 1-2 inches long and is found in characteristic clusters around the ileocecal valve (Fig 10).

Concentrations of *A perfoliata* result in severe ulcerations of the mucosa. A few tapeworms may be present without causing definite clinical signs; however, heavier infections cause chronic

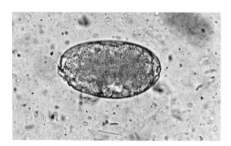

Figure 8. A trichostrongyle egg from fresh feces. (350X)

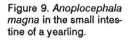

Figure 9. *Anoplocephala magna* in the small intestine of a yearling.

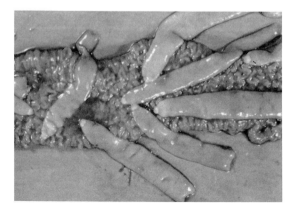

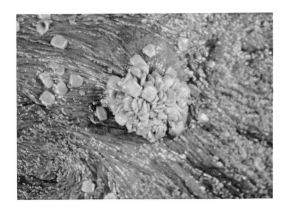

Figure 10. Cluster of *Anoplocephala perfoliata* at the ileocecal valve in a yearling.

unthriftiness, intermittent colic and diarrhea. Perforation of the cecum or occlusion of the ileocecal sphincter has resulted in death. As a clinical entity, tapeworm infections in horses are usually not a widespread problem. When it does occur, one or several young horses become acutely ill or are found dead.

Life Cycle: The life cycle of these tapeworms involves an intermediate host, orbatid mites, which exist as free-living forms on pastures. The prevalence of tapeworm infections in horses is related to geographic distribution of the mites. Development of cysticercoids in the mites takes 2-4 months. Adult tapeworms develop 2 months after horses ingest the mites.

Diagnosis: Tapeworm infection is diagnosed by finding the typical angular eggs in a fecal flotation (Fig 11). The discharge of proglottids in light infections is sporadic. Therefore, a single fecal examination may fail to disclose tapeworm infection.

Lungworms

Dictyocaulus

The lungworm, *Dictyocaulus arnfieldi,* is prevalent in donkeys, considered to be the normal host. Horses pastured with donkeys have a greater possibility of infection, though the incidence in horses is usually low. Infected animals may be asymptomatic or may have a persistent cough.

Life Cycle: The life cycle of this parasite is indirect. Earthworms are the intermediate hosts.

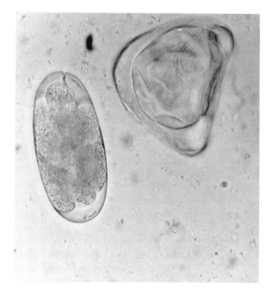

Figure 11. Angular *Anoplocephala* egg (right) in contrast to a strongyle egg (left).

Figure 12. An egg of *Dictyocaulus arnfieldi*. (350X)

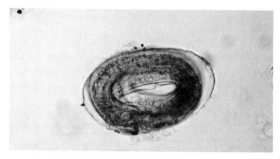

Diagnosis: Dictyocaulus arnfieldi produces a larvated egg; however, its egg is larger and more oval than *Habronema* eggs and the contained larva is more coiled (Fig 12). *Dictyocaulus arnfieldi* eggs are often already hatched in fresh feces. Typical spiked-tail larvae may be found in fresh feces by performing fecal smears, flotations, or the Baermann technique. The Baermann technique produces the best results.

Liver Flukes

Fasciola

Fasciola hepatica is the common liver fluke of ruminants. If cattle and sheep in fluke-enzootic areas are grazed on the same pastures as horses, horses can become infected. Clinical signs include anorexia, weight loss, abdominal pain, anemia and diarrhea.

Diagnosis: Fasciola hepatica eggs are large (130-150 µ), yellowish brown and smooth shelled, with an operculum at one end (Fig 13). Because these eggs do not float in ordinary flotation solution, fecal sedimentation is the preferred method of examining feces for eggs.

Eyeworms

Thelazia

Thelazia species, or eyeworms, are roundworms that live on the eyes of horses and other domestic animals. The adults are milky white and 7-17 mm long. They reside under the eyelids, particularly the third eyelid, and on the surface of the eyeball.

Life Cycle: Like stomach worms, these spirurid nematodes require an intermediate host in their life cycle. The most common intermediate host is the face fly, *Musca autumnalis*. The life cycle takes about 4 months to complete. The highest rate of infection is in horses under 4 years of age.

Diagnosis: The infection usually causes no clinical signs. Larvae may be evident in lacrimal fluid. A local ophthalmic anesthetic may be applied to the eye for examination, which may reveal adult worms.

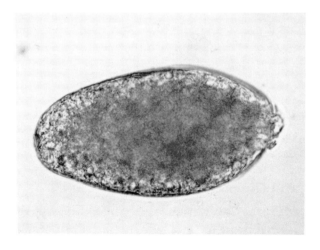

Figure 13. An egg of *Fasciola hepatica*. (350X)

Filarial Nematodes

Onchocerca, Setaria and *Dirofilaria*

Two filarial nematodes sometimes seen in horses are *Onchocerca cervicalis,* the neck threadworm, and *Setaria equina.* *Onchocerca cervicalis* invades the ligamentum nuchae and produces microfilariae that migrate to the superficial areas of the skin. Skin lesions can be scraped or biopsied to demonstrate the microfilariae.

Setaria equina is a parasite of the abdominal cavity of equine species. Aberrant larvae occasionally cause lumbar paralysis, also called "cerebrospinal nematodiasis" or "kumri," which is usually fatal.

Dirofilaria immitis, the heartworm of dogs, produces microfilariae and occasionally is found in horses. The clinical significance of heartworm infection in horses is unknown, though pneumonic and arteriosclerotic lesions have been found in infected horses at necropsy.

Protozoa

Eimeria

Eimeria leuckarti is the only intestinal coccidian of horses in the United States. It usually is found in horses less than a year old. Infections are usually asymptomatic and self-limiting, and horses rapidly become immune to further infection.

Diagnosis: Oocysts are passed in feces. Compared to oocysts of many other species of coccidia, this oocyst is very large (75-90 μ long). It is thick walled and dark brown, with a distinct micropyle (opening) at its narrow end (Fig 14). Regular flotation solutions do not float these larger oocysts. Though such solutions as saturated sodium nitrate (1:360) and saturated sugar (1:320) may float these oocysts, fecal sedimentation is probably a better method to detect this parasite (see Chapter 2).

Tritrichomonas and *Giardia*

Tritrichomonas equi is a flagellate protozoan that is considered to be a normal inhabitant of the large intestine of horses.

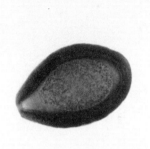

Figure 14. An oocyst of *Eimeria leuckarti*. (350X)

Giardia equi is a flagellate protozoan of low incidence in horses. It invades the small intestine and causes chronic diarrhea. Normal flotation techniques rarely detect this parasite, but a 33% zinc sulfate (1:180) flotation solution can float the *Giardia* cysts.

Sarcocystis and Klossiella

Sarcocystis species are sporadically found in the asexual or schizogonous stage of development in horses. This stage can invade the central nervous system, producing a condition called equine protozoal myeloencephalitis. This disease most commonly affects Standardbreds and Thoroughbreds. Clinical signs are similar to those seen in "wobblers": ataxia, weakness, stumbling, muscle wasting and disorientation.

Klossiella equi is a nonpathogenic coccidian that can infect the kidneys of horses. Oocysts can occasionally be found in urine.

References

1. Bello, in Mansmann and McAllister: *Equine Medicine and Surgery.* 3rd ed. American Veterinary Publications, Goleta, CA, 1982.

2. Lichenfels: *Proc Helm Soc Wash*, 1975.

3. Ogbourne: Commonwealth Agri Bureau, Bucks, England, 1978.

4. Bello *et al: Proc 20th Ann Mtg AAEP*, 1974. p 97.

5. Clayton and Duncan: *Res Vet Sci* 26:383, 1979.

6. Clayton and Duncan: *Intl J Parasitol* 9:285, 1979.

7. Lyons *et al: J Parasitol* 59:780, 1973.

8. Greer *et al: J Parasitol* 60:466, 1974.

6

External Parasites
of Horses

L.J. Ackerman

Mites

Sarcoptes scabiei

Sarcoptic mange is a reportable disease caused by the scabies mite, *Sarcoptes scabiei* var *equi*, a burrowing mite that causes intense pruritus. The condition is contagious and people in contact with infested horses may acquire the mites, though the mites have difficulty reproducing on people. The female mite burrows into the epidermis and the life cycle is completed in 10-17 days. The mites may persist in the environment for up to 3 weeks.

Clinical Signs: These mites prefer certain areas on the body and are most commonly recovered from around the head and neck. The initial lesions include papules, vesicles and hair loss but may progress to severe generalized scaling and crusting dermatitis, with excoriations and lichenification associated with intense pruritus.

Diagnosis: Diagnosis is by the history, clinical signs of intense pruritus, multiple skin scrapings and possibly biopsy. The mites are exceedingly difficult to recover and it is not unusual for multiple skin scrapings to be negative. Similarly, biopsies are only informative if a section of mite actually appears on the microscope slide.

Areas with erythematous, papular rash and crusts should be scraped. Multiple skin scrapings are needed to demonstrate sarcoptic mites. Adult sarcoptic mites are oval and about 200-400 μ in diameter, with 4 pairs of legs (Fig 1). Females have long, unsegmented pedicles, with suckers on 2 pairs of legs. Males have long, unsegmented pedicles, with suckers on 3 pairs of legs. The anus is located at the caudal end of the body. The 8-legged nymphs of sarcoptic mites are smaller than the adults. The 6-legged larva lacks a caudal pair of legs. The eggs of sarcoptic mites are oval (Fig 2).

Chorioptes equi

Chorioptic mange, caused by the host-specific mite *Chorioptes equi*, is uncommon in horses. The mites have a 2- to 3-week life cycle, do not affect people and can live away from their host in the environment for a few days.

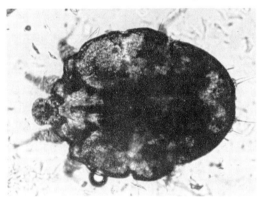

Figure 1. *Sarcoptes scabiei.* These mites are oval and have long, unsegmented pedicles, with suckers on several pairs of legs. The anus is terminal.

Figure 2. Eggs from sarcoptic mites are oval. (Courtesy of R. Bell, Texas A&M Univ)

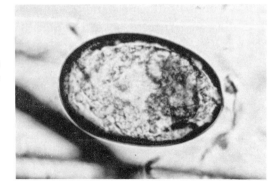

Clinical Signs: Chorioptic mange typically affects the distal limbs and perineum, causing pruritic maculopapular to papulocrustous dermatitis. When only the distal limbs are affected, chorioptic mange is difficult to differentiate from other causes of pastern dermatitis (grease heel). This presentation is more commonly seen in Draft horses and others with feathered fetlocks.

Diagnosis: Diagnosis is by the history, clinical signs and skin scrapings to demonstrate the mites, larvae and eggs (Fig 3). Chorioptic mites are about 400 μ long. Females have short, unsegmented pedicles, with suckers on 3 of their 4 pairs of legs (Fig 4). Males have short, unsegmented pedicles, with suckers on all 4 pairs of legs.

Psoroptes equi

Psoroptic mange is a reportable disease caused by the predominantly host-specific mite *Psoroptes equi*. The mites do not burrow or parasitize people, have a 10- to 14-day life cycle and can live away from their host in the environment for up to 3 weeks. These mites are surface-dwelling parasites that feed on epidermal debris.

Clinical Signs: The clinical presentation is usually a pruritic maculopapular to papulocrustous eruption, predominantly of the mane and tail region. Pruritus is variable but usually marked. The forehead and ear canals may also be affected, and

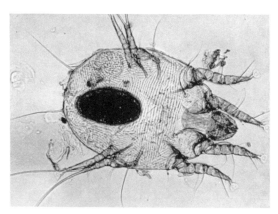

Figure 3. A female *Chorioptes* mite containing an egg. (Courtesy of R. Bell, Texas A&M Univ)

head shaking and rubbing may be a significant component of the clinical presentation. It has also been proposed that *P cuniculi* and *P hippotis* may affect the ear canals of horses.

Diagnosis: Diagnosis is by the history, clinical signs, otoscopy and skin scrapings to demonstrate the mites, larvae and eggs. Psoroptic mites are easily demonstrated in scrapings from the edge of the lesions. The adult mites are about 800 μ long and may be seen grossly or with the aid of a hand magnifier (Fig 5). Magnification under low power (10X objective) is necessary for specific identification. Both male and female mites have long, segmented pedicles on 3 of their 4 pairs of legs.

Chigger Mites

The larvae of chiggers (*eg, Eutrombicula alfreddugesi, Trombicula batatas, Trombicula spendens* and perhaps *Walchia americana*) usually parasitize rodents, birds, snakes and lizards in wooded areas. The adults are free living and do not feed on animals. Animals roaming through infested environments may acquire the parasitic larval forms. This problem is more prevalent in the late summer and fall.

Clinical Signs: The bites of chigger mites are quite irritating and pruritic, with most bites occurring in the region of the head and legs. This results in a maculopapular eruption in those areas.

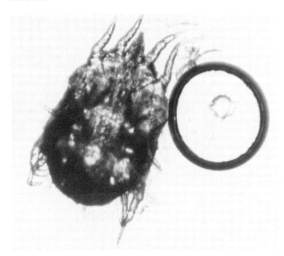

Figure 4. *Psoroptes* mite taken from the ear of a horse. The circular structure on the right is an air bubble.

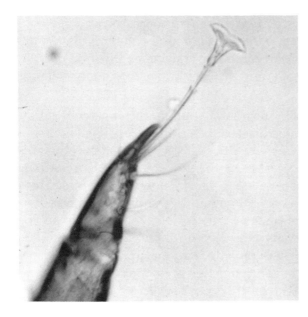

Figure 5. *Psoroptes* mites have long, unsegmented pedicles, with suckers on 3 of their 4 pairs of legs (Courtesy of R. Bell, Texas A&M Univ)

Diagnosis: Diagnosis is by the history, (exposure to forests, late summer or fall), clinical examination (larvae may occasionally be seen as orange dots) and skin scrapings (to reveal larvae).

Demodex equi

Demodex equi is a mite that is a normal resident of equine skin, living within the hair follicles and only appearing on the skin surface when travelling between follicles. Demodicid mites of one species or another are present in small numbers on the skin of all normal mammals, including people and are therefore considered noncontagious. In these small numbers they do not cause any disease, but simply feed on debris within the hair follicles. The life cycle requires 20-35 days to complete.

Demodicosis or demodectic mange is generally considered a rare disease of horses. If *Demodex* mites are present on all normal animals, why do some animals develop mite-related disease (mange) and most do not? Animals with demodectic mange may have an inherited or acquired immune defect that fails to keep the mite numbers in check. The result is a demodectic mite population explosion. Though stress or corticosteroid use may be a triggering mechanism for clinical episodes, the

mite themselves, once their numbers increase, produce substances that further suppress the immune system. This secondary immunosuppression can be reversed once the mite population is eliminated, but any primary inherited immune defect
cannot be corrected.

Clinical Signs: The degree of immunoincompetence deter-
mines the extent of skin disease. The skin disease itself is caused
by the mites effectively crowding out the hairs within the hair
follicles, eventually destroying the hair follicle. If the contents
of the follicle (*eg,* hair debris, bacteria, mites) are released into
the dermis, infection and inflammation result. The redness, hair
loss and infection are what we refer to as demodectic mange. The
generalized form is characterized by large areas of hair loss,
redness, scaling and papulopustular dermatitis. Nodular dermatitis occasionally is evident, but this presentation is more common in goats and cattle than in horses. Areas affected most often
are the head, neck, withers and legs. The mites may be more
numerous during the summer.

Diagnosis: Diagnosis of demodicosis is not difficult. Skin
scrapings are performed by removing the top layers of epidermis
by scraping with a scalpel blade or similar instrument and
viewing the characteristic mites, larvae and eggs under the
microscope. The procedure can be facilitated by squeezing the
skin before scraping to express the mites from the hair follicles.
Alternatively, if scrapings are not done, the mites are easily seen
within the hair follicles on biopsy specimens. *Demodex* mites are
elongated, with short, stubby legs (Fig 6). Adults and nymphs
have 8 legs, and larvae have 6 legs. The adults are about 250 μ
long. The eggs are fusiform (Fig 7).

Straw-Itch Mites

Pyemotes tritici, the straw-itch mite, normally parasitizes
larvae of grain insects. Horses may become infested from contaminated hay fed from overhead racks. People may be infested.

Clinical Signs: The maculopapular papulocrustous eruption
that ensues is predominantly nonpruritic. Most of the eruption
is seen on the head, neck and chest.

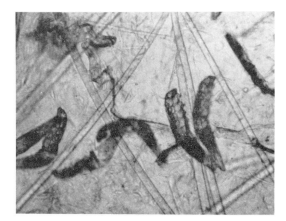

Figure 6. *Demodex* mites are elongated and have short stubby legs.

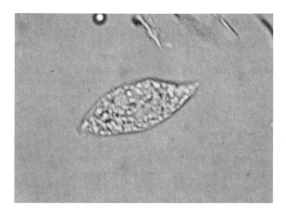

Figure 7. *Demodex* eggs are fusiform.

Infested people are often quite pruritic and lesions include erythema, macules, papules and urticarial plaques.

Diagnosis: Diagnosis is by the history, clinical examination, feed analysis and skin scrapings.

Ticks

Ticks are members of the spider family (arachnids) and are blood-sucking parasites capable of transmitting a variety of protozoal (*eg,* babesiosis, anaplasmosis), rickettsial (*eg,* Rocky Mountain spotted fever, ehrlichiosis), viral (*eg,* St. Louis encephalitis) and bacterial (*eg,* tularemia) diseases, in addition to dermatologic disorders, paralysis and anemia. Ticks are responsible for transmission of the newly recognized "Lyme disease."

Tick-related dermatoses are most commonly seen in the spring and summer.

There are 2 major families of ticks. Soft ticks (*eg, Otobius megnini, Ornithodorus coriaecus*) have no shield, and the larvae and nymphs are parasitic. Those of *Otobius megnini* usually parasitize the external ear canal of horses (Fig 8). These ticks infest barns, sheds and other areas where animals are found. Hard ticks (*eg, Dermacentor, Ixodes, Ambylomma*) are the most common ticks affecting horses. The larvae, nymphs and adults are all parasitic. Hard ticks live outdoors and attach to passing animals.

Clinical Signs: Clinical signs include a maculopapular eruption, otitis externa and papularnodular dermatitis consisting of small nodules, or, in the case of a hypersensitivity reaction, urticarial plaques.

Diagnosis: Diagnosis is by clinical signs and visualization of the ticks.

Lice

Lice are wingless insects that are host-specific and have adapted to parasitize only certain species. They are transmitted by direct contact or by contaminated objects, such as brushes,

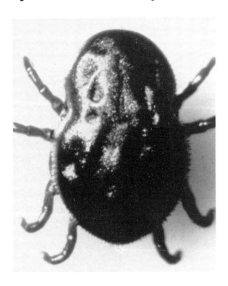

Figure 8. *Otobius megnini* nymph has leathery consistency. (Courtesy of Extension Vet Med, Univ California)

blankets and tack. The entire life cycle, from egg (nit) to nymph to adult, requires about 3 weeks. Adult lice can survive away from the host only for a short period. There are 2 different types of lice. Biting lice (*eg, Damalinia equi*) feed on epidermal debris and hair. Sucking lice (*eg, Hematopinus asini*) pierce the skin and feed on tissue fluids.

Clinical Signs: Infested animals have a dull, dry coat with hair loss, scales and crusts. Adult lice and nits can normally be seen on the haircoat. Animals infested with sucking lice may also be anemic because of blood loss.

Diagnosis: Diagnosis is not difficult, as the lice can usually be seen on the haircoat with careful examination (Fig 9).

Fleas

Fleas are wingless insects, 1.0-2.5 mm long, with laterally compressed bodies and mouth parts structured for puncturing

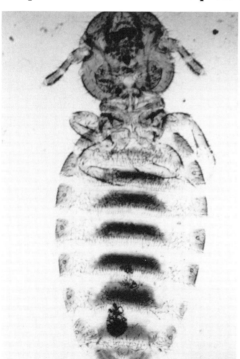

Figure 9. *Damalinia equi*, the biting louse of horses.

the skin to suck blood. The major species infesting horses are *Tunga penetrans* and *Echidnophaga gallinacea.*

Clinical signs of flea infestation include pruritus, excoriations, papules, crusting and resultant alopecia. Diagnosis is based on the history, clinical signs and visualization of the fleas (see Chapter 4).

Flies

Flies undergo a complete metamorphosis in their life cycles, from egg to larva, to pupa to adult. Some flies may cause dermatologic problems from their irritating bites, hypersensitivity reactions, laying eggs within existing sores (myiasis), or by completing their life cycles under the skin (warbles).

Stomoxys calcitrans

Fly bites, especially those of the stable fly *Stomoxys calcitrans*, can be very irritating and may bleed freely. In addition, *Stomoxys calcitrans* can transmit *Habronema* spp, which can result in cutaneous habronemiasis. The flies lay their eggs in rotting organic matter, such as hay or manure. The life cycle is complete in 30-60 days.

Clinical Signs: Horses may be bitten anywhere, but the flies prefer areas around the head and ears, topline, ventral midline and legs. The lesions appear in a maculopapular eruption as little red bumps on the skin, with scaling, crusting and hair loss, with or without associated bleeding.

Diagnosis: Diagnosis is based on the history and clinical signs, and may be supported by biopsy.

Culicoides

Culicoides flies or gnats are primarily active from dusk to dawn, especially during the warmer months (Fig 10). They are annoying to horses and serve as intermediate hosts for *Onchocerca cervicalis.* These flies have 2 basic feeding patterns: dorsal and ventral. Dorsal-feeding species of *Culicoides* feed about the mane and tail, and may cause a hypersensitivity reaction called by a variety of names, including Queensland itch, summer itch,

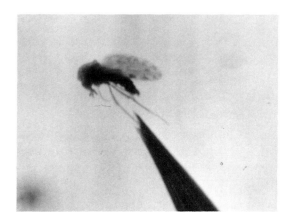

Figure 10. *Culicoides varii-pennis*, with its mottled wings, is one of the main causes of "summer itch."

kasen, dhobie itch and muck itch. Ventral-feeding species of *Culicoides* cause ventral midline dermatitis.

Clinical Signs: The clinical presentation is usually quite consistent. Horses are often between 1 and 5 years of age when first affected. There is an obvious seasonal trend. It is usually seen in horses kept outside and only a few horses in a group are affected. Lesions, which include scaling, hair loss, crusting, ulceration and lichenification associated with pruritus, may be exclusively dorsal (including "rat tail") or ventral.

Diagnosis: Diagnosis may be aided by the history, clinical examination, complete blood counts (eosinophilia), biopsy (eosinophilic perivascular dermatitis) and allergy testing with *Culicoides* antigen.

Lyperosia irritans

The horn fly, *Lyperosia (Hematobia) irritans*, requires fresh feces in which to lay eggs. They are also a vector for *Stephanofilaria stilesi*, a filarial nematode of cattle.

Clinical Signs: The flies have piercing mouthparts and can inflict considerable damage, resulting in pruritus, excoriations and crusting. In the horse they are responsible for seasonal focal ventral midline dermatosis centered about the umbilicus.

Diagnosis: Diagnosis is based on the history, clinical signs and biopsy findings of eosinophilic perivascular dermatitis.

Miscellaneous Flies

Musca autumnalis, the face fly, feeds on oculonasal secretions and is much more a problem of cattle than horses. They require fresh feces in which to lay their eggs. The problems caused are related to annoyance and irritation, though they are a vector of *Moraxella bovis*, one of the causes of pinkeye.

Horseflies (*Tabanus* spp) and deer flies (*Chrysops* spp) are large flies that can do considerable damage with their aggressive biting. They also can transmit equine infectious anemia, anthrax, anaplasmosis and trypanosomiasis. Treatment is difficult but may be attempted with residual insecticides or heavy applications of pyrethrins or pyrethroids. The flies require water to complete their life cycle and are most active on hot summer days.

Black flies (*Simulium* spp) are particularly active in summer months, especially in areas with fresh, running water (Fig 11). They cause painful and often bleeding bites, especially on the head, ears, ventrum and legs. In addition to their vicious bites, they may cause anemia when present in large numbers and also may transmit the filarial nematode *Onchocerca cervicalis*.

Warbles (*Hypoderma* spp) occasionally infest horses, though they are more commonly found in cattle (see Chapter 8). The flies lay their eggs on the haircoat. The larvae then penetrate the skin and migrate, and by spring create a nodule and often a breathing pore on the dorsum. Because the horse is not a definitive host for the parasite, the life cycle is often not completed.

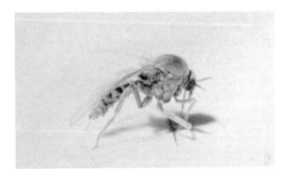

Figure 11. The black fly, *Simulium*. Note the humped thorax and transparent wings.

Some flies lay eggs in organic matter or in any open wound on a horse's skin. The eggs hatch in a day or so and larvae (maggots) begin to feed on damaged tissue. Most larvae only feed on dead tissue and do not invade living skin. Toxins released from the larvae, however, may further damage surrounding tissue to the extent that it is then suitable for continued feeding. In such areas as the southwestern United States, where the screwworm fly (*Callitroga hominivorax*) is still present, larvae should be collected in 70% ethyl alcohol and sent to authorities for identification.

Mosquitoes

Mosquito bites are not only a nuisance but also may transmit viral and protozoal diseases. The major species affecting horses are *Aedes* spp, *Anopheles* spp and *Culex* spp. A source of water is required for egg laying.

Clinical signs include macules, papules, wheals and erythema, with variable pruritus and pain. Diagnosis is based on the history and clinical signs.

Helminths

Habronema

Habronema nematodes have a worldwide distribution but are most important in moist, warm climates where the intermediate hosts are prevalent. *Habronema* adults develop in the gastric mucosa. The eggs are passed and hatch in manure. Larvae are ingested in maggots, which mature into flies. When the flies feed on the horse's lips, the *Habronema* larvae pass through the proboscis of the fly, are swallowed by the horse and reach maturity in the horse's stomach. Horses may also become infected when they swallow dead flies.

Cutaneous habronemiasis (summer sores) is caused by aberrant deposition of *Habronema* larvae in wounds. The lesions consist of excessive granulation tissue containing small, yellow, caseous areas (granules), most commonly located on the distal extremities, male genitalia and medial canthus.

Diagnosis of cutaneous habronemiasis is based on clinical signs and skin biopsies. Attempts to demonstrate the larvae in skin scrapings or granules are usually unrewarding.

Onchocerca cervicalis

The microfilaria of the adult filarid nematode *Onchocerca cervicalis* causes recurrent dermatitis and is thought to cause periodic ophthalmia in horses. Adults live in the ligamentum nuchae in the neck of horses. Females produce microfilariae, which migrate to the dermis via connective tissue. *Onchocerca cervicalis* is transmitted by the bites of *Culicoides* spp, known as biting midges, punkies or no-see-ums. The microfilariae are picked up by the *Culicoides* when the flies feed on a horse's belly and develop in the fly into infective larvae. When the fly bites another horse, larvae are injected into connective tissue and develop into adults during migration to the ligamentum nuchae.

Lesions of cutaneous onchocerciasis consist of patchy alopecia, scaling on the head, neck, shoulders and ventral midline, sometimes with intense pruritus.

Many infected horses are asymptomatic. The microfilariae concentrate in certain areas, with the ventral midline the most common area of concentrations of microfilariae in normal horses. Because over 90% of normal horses are probably infested with *O cervicalis*, detection of microfilariae in the skin of the ventral midline is not diagnostic of cutaneous onchocerciasis. However, the presence of microfilariae in diseased skin in areas other than the ventral midline is highly suggestive, though not diagnostic, of cutaneous onchocerciasis.

Onchocerca microfilariae may be demonstrated by the following procedure. After clipping and a surgical scrub, a 6-mm punch biopsy is obtained. With a single-edged razor blade or scalpel blade, half of the tissue is minced in a small amount of preservative-free physiologic saline on a glass slide and is allowed to stand for 10-15 minutes. Drying of the specimen is prevented by placing the slide in a covered chamber with a small amount of saline (Fig 12). The slide is then examined under a low-power (10X) objective. Because the translucent microfilariae may be difficult to see, low-intensity light and high contrast (achieved

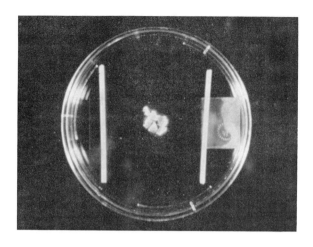

Figure 12. *Onchocerca* preparation.

by lowering the condenser) are essential. Live microfilariae are identified by their vigorous swimming movement in the saline at the periphery of the tissue. *Onchocerca cervicalis* microfilariae are slender and 207-240 μ long (Fig 13). The other half of the biopsy should be submitted for routine histopathologic examination.

Pelodera strongyloides

Pelodera strongyloides is a free-living parasite often found in organic matter, such as damp hay or straw. The larvae may actively penetrate a horse's skin during periods of direct contact, such as when these materials are used as bedding.

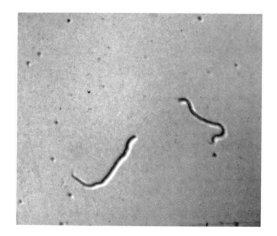

Figure 13. *Onchocerca* microfilariae at the periphery of a piece of minced skin.

Clinical Signs: Infestation with *Pelodera strongyloides* can result in a maculopapular eruption that is worse in areas of direct contact with the source of parasites (*eg,* hay, straw).

Diagnosis: Diagnosis is based on the history and clinical signs, and confirmed by finding characteristic larvae on skin scrapings (Fig 14).

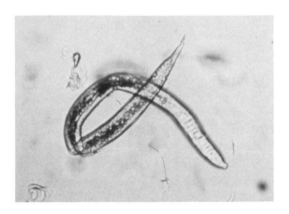

Figure 14. *Pelodera strongyloides* larva. (Courtesy of J. MacDonald, Auburn Univ)

7

Internal Parasites of Food Animals

W.F. Wade and S.M. Gaafar

Parasites of Ruminants

Eimeria

Eimeria is a coccidian that may cause diarrhea in ruminants. Many different species of *Eimeria* parasitize ruminants. The oocysts range in size from 10-50 μ, depending on their species. The oocysts can be partially differentiated by size and appearance (Fig 1).

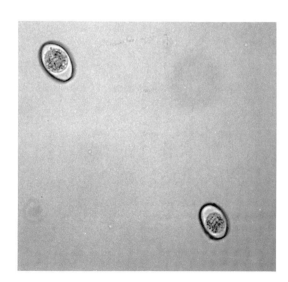

Figure 1. Two oocysts of *Eimeria* from fresh goat feces. (350X)

Cryptosporidium

Cryptosporidium bovis is another coccidian parasite that may produce severe diarrhea in newborn calves. The size of the oocyst (4-6 μ) makes detection in fecal samples difficult. Oocysts are more often found by microscopic examination of intestinal mucosal cells. Using fecal flotation, you may be able to see the small, pale oval bodies with a darker central area. The preserved fecal sample is then best sent to an animal disease diagnostic laboratory to confirm the diagnosis.

Fasciola hepatica

Fasciola hepatica is a liver fluke of ruminants. It is the most important trematode of livestock in the world. It is an increasing problem as new dams, irrigation projects and improved water facilities are developed and provide new habitats for the snail intermediate hosts. Acute liver fluke infection causes high mortality in sheep, while the chronic form results in substantial losses in cattle and sheep.

In the United States, *F hepatica* occurs primarily in the Gulf Coast and western states, while *F gigantica* is found in Hawaii. *Fascioloides magna*, the American fluke, is an additional problem in the Gulf Coast states, Great Lakes region and northwestern states, where cattle and sheep share pastures with deer, elk or moose, the natural hosts.

Diagnosis: The eggs of *F hepatica* and *F magna* are large (130-150 μ), yellowish brown and smooth shelled, with an oper-

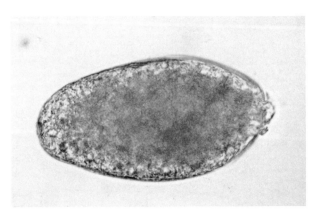

Figure 2. An egg of *Fasciola hepatica*. (350X)

culum at one end (Fig 2). Because these eggs do not float in ordinary flotation solution, fecal sedimentation is the preferred method of examining feces for these eggs.

Dicrocoelium dendriticum

Dicrocoelium dendriticum, the lancet liver fluke, is restricted to areas of New York state. It has small (36-45 μ), brown eggs. The shell is thick and has a barely visible operculum at one end (Fig 3). These eggs are best seen by fecal sediment examination.

Paramphistomum microbothroides

These rumen flukes appear to be of minor economic significance in the United States, though heavy infections can cause severe enteritis and mortality in cattle and occasionally in sheep. *Paramphistomum microbothroides* is the most common rumen fluke of cattle in the United States.

Moniezia

Moniezia spp are tapeworms of ruminants. Their eggs may be spherical, but usually the thick shell is pressed into a triangular or quadrangular shape (Fig 4). The egg contains a hexacanth embryo surrounded by a pyriform apparatus and is 50-90 μ wide. A less common type of ruminant tapeworm is *Thysanosoma actinioides*, the fringe tapeworm, which produces egg packets, each containing several hexacanth embryos.

The eggs of ruminant tapeworms may be seen on fecal flotation, but disruption of a tapeworm segment from the feces and examination of its contents is a better method for identification.

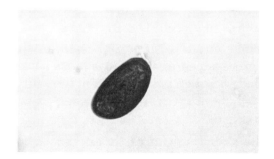

Figure 3. An egg of *Dicrocoelium dendriticum*. (350X)

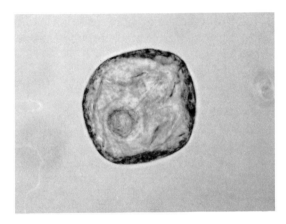

Figure 4. An egg of *Moniezia* sp. (350X)

Trichostrongyles

Worms of the genera *Hemonchus, Trichostrongylus, Cooperia, Oesophagostomum, Bunostomum, Ostertagia* and *Chabertia* inhabit the abomasum or intestines of ruminants. They are the most significant group of internal parasites in cattle and sheep, and can produce severe disease in heavy infections. Under adverse environmental conditions, many of these parasites become dormant for up to 6 months, and resume development when conditions are again favorable. This phenomenon is called "hypobiosis" or "arrested development," and creates considerable problems in parasite control.

Diagnosis: All trichostrongyles produce eggs that are similar in appearance. Though there are some differences in size and shape, it is usually impractical to attempt to specifically identify the species of eggs. Trichostrongyle larvae hatched from the eggs in fecal culture may be used for identification, but that also is difficult. The eggs are all oval, thin shelled and 70-120 μ long, with contents divided into 4 or more cells (Fig 5).

Hemonchus: The common name of this worm, the barberpole worm, is derived from its gross appearance. Being a blood sucker, its intestine is blood filled and when twisted around the white ovary and uterus of the female, it gives the appearance of an old-fashioned barber pole (Fig 6).

Hemonchus lives in the abomasum of cattle and sheep in warmer climates. The blood-sucking feeding habits of this par-

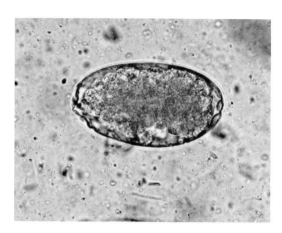

Figure 5. A trichostrongyle egg from fresh bovine feces. (350X)

asite can result in significant anemia in calves and lambs, with little or no diarrhea. Other clinical signs include anorexia, weight loss, submandibular edema ("bottle jaw") and, in heavy infections, death.

Ostertagia ostertagi: The brown stomach worm is the most pathogenic economically important parasite of cattle and sheep in the United States.

Ostertagia parasitizes the abomasal gastric glands. Major lesions occur when worms emerge from these glands and enter the lumen of the abomasum. Nodules form around parasitized gastric glands, causing loss of HCl-producing cells. In severe cases, the nodules coalesce to form a hyperplastic mucosa that

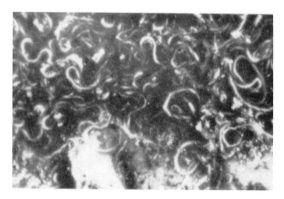

Figure 6. Numerous *Hemonchus* worms on the mucosal surface of the abomasum. Some of the female worms have a striped appearance, resembling a barber pole.

is described as having a "Morocco leather" appearance. Diarrhea is a consistent finding. Heavy worm burdens are usually fatal.

Trichostrongylus: The abomasal worm, *T axei*, occurs in cattle and sheep throughout North America. It causes an acute disease characterized by anorexia and blackish diarrhea, or, more commonly, a chronic wasting disease.

Several species of *Trichostrongylus* inhabit the intestine of ruminants. In large numbers or in combination with other internal parasites, they can pose significant problems. Though *T colubriformis* and *T longispicularis* are primarily parasites of sheep, they have been reported in cattle. The pathogenesis of the infection is not fully understood, and infected animals may show few signs. However, in some cases, anorexia, diarrhea and even death may occur.

Cooperia: This parasite is limited to specific geographic areas usually defined by climate. These worms penetrate the mucosa of the small intestine and suck blood. Heavy infections in calves cause serious disease and death.

Oesophagostomum radiatum: The nodular worm takes its name from the lesion it induces in the large intestine. Ingested infective larvae penetrate small and large intestinal mucosa. In primary infections, small nodules form around the larvae in the mucosa. The nodules resolve when the larvae return to the gut lumen to develop into adults. With repeated infections, the nodules increase to over 1 cm in diameter and are filled with caseous material. Often the nodules coalesce to form large caseous lesions that may rupture into the abdominal cavity.

Though generally considered to be a warm weather parasite, *Oesophagostomum* is found throughout the United States. Acute clinical signs are characterized by anorexia, weakness and black, fetid diarrhea. The more chronic form causes intermittent diarrhea that later becomes continuous, with a black or dark green color and a strong odor.

Bunostomum phlebotomum: This hookworm of cattle is a voracious blood feeder. The third-stage larvae of the small intestinal parasite enter the body by penetrating intact skin or being ingested. Adults attach to the intestinal mucosa and suck blood (Fig 7).

Bunostomum is a warm-weather parasite and does not survive well in cold conditions. It is a particular problem in calves confined to a small area.

Nematodirus: Nematodirus is the thread-necked intestinal worm of ruminants. This parasite is also considered to belong to the trichostrongyle group; however, its egg has a distinctive appearance and larger size than other trichostrongyle eggs. *Nematodirus* eggs are football shaped, contain 2-8 dark cells and are comparatively large (150-230 μ) (Fig 8).

Hypobiosis: All the above parasites, to a greater or lesser degree, can enter into a state called "hypobiosis" or "arrested development." This is a condition in which larvae remain dormant in the host body and resistant to most anthelmintics. This period of inactivity is associated with times of adverse environmental conditions, such as cold temperatures in the north or hot, arid summer conditions in the south. Hypobiosis is a survival mechanism whereby the parasite can survive safely in an inhospitable environment and emerge at a more favorable time.

During hypobiosis, which can last up to 6 months, the parasites do not produce eggs; therefore, fecal examinations give no indication of the number of parasites present in the animal. An animal with a negative fecal examination can, in fact, have a heavy parasite infection. Further, the emergence of parasites

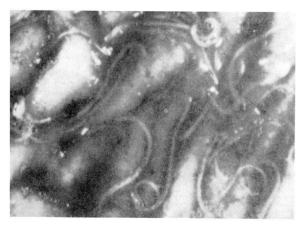

Figure 7. Closeup view of duodenal mucosa with numerous *Bunostomum* adults.

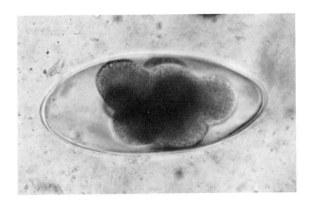

Figure 8. An egg of
Nematodirus sp. (350X)

from their hypobiotic state serves as a source of pasture contamination on what are often parasite-free pastures.

Trichuris

The whipworms of cattle and sheep (*Trichuris* spp) have eggs similar in size and shape to those of *Trichuris vulpis* (see Chapter 3, Fig 5).

Strongyloides

Larvated eggs seen in fresh ruminant feces are likely to be those of *Strongyloides*. These eggs are similar in size and shape to those of *Strongyloides ransomi* of pigs (Fig 19).

Dictyocaulus

This slender nematode, known as the lungworm, is found in the trachea and bronchi of cattle and measures up to 8 cm in length. Clinical signs include coughing and labored breathing, with eventual development of bronchitis. Heavily infected calves can die as soon as 3 weeks after infection. It causes serious disease in cattle in areas of high rainfall and moderate temperature. Infection in sheep, caused by *Dictyocaulus filaria*, is not as severe. The free-living stages can overwinter on pasture or in a state of arrested development in the host.

Diagnosis: Eggs of *Dictyocaulus* of ruminants hatch during passage through the intestines, so that larvae are seen in the feces. *Dictyocaulus viviparus* produces larvae containing many dark intestinal granules. Their tail ends in a blunt point and they are 390-450 µ long (Fig 9). Larvae of *Dictyocaulus filaria* of sheep have similar granules and a blunt tail, but have a small knob on the cranial end. *Dictyocaulus filaria* larvae range in length from 550 µ to 580 µ. Lungworm larvae may be seen on fecal flotation, but the preferred method of examination is the Baermann technique (described in Chapter 2).

Muellerius capillaris

Muellerius capillaris is a lungworm of sheep and goats. This larva does not have the dark granules seen in *Dictyocaulus* larvae and has a pronounced kink in its tail (Fig 10). The Baermann technique is the preferred method of fecal exam.

Anaplasma

Anaplasma is a rickettsial blood parasite of ruminants. In stained thin blood smears, these rickettsiae appear as small red or dark-red dots inside the RBC (Fig 11). *Anaplasma marginale* is located near the cell wall, while *A centrale* is located centrally in the cell.

Trypanosoma

Trypanosoma, a protozoan blood parasite of ruminants, has a long, narrow body with a dark nucleus, a flagellum and a

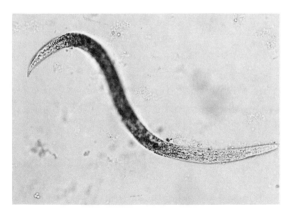

Figure 9. A larva of *Dictyocaulus viviparus*. (225X)

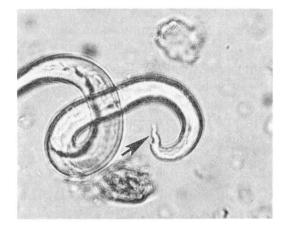

Figure 10. A larva of *Muellerius capillaris.* Note the kink in the tail (arrow). (560X)

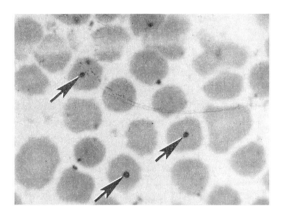

Figure 11. *Anaplasma* sp (arrows) in a thin blood smear from a cow. (1400X)

sail-like undulating membrane (Fig 12). They are seen between RBC in a thin blood smear.

Thelazia

Thelazia spp are roundworms that live on the eyes of several species of domestic animals, including cattle, sheep, goats, horses, dogs and cats. The adult parasites are milky white and 7-17 mm long, and reside under the eyelids, particularly the third eyelid, and on the surface of the eyeball. Diagnosis is by anesthetizing the eye with a local ophthalmologic anesthetic and directly examining the eye for the parasites.

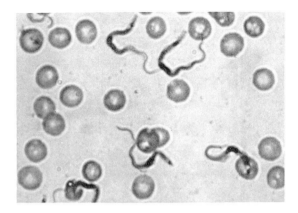

Figure 12. *Trypanosoma* in a bovine blood smear. (1400X)

Tritrichomonas foetus

Tritrichomonas foetus is a protozoan parasite of the reproductive tract of cattle. They reside in the prepuce of infected bulls and the vagina, cervix and uterus of infected cows.

Tritrichomonas foetus is pear shaped and 10-25 μ long, with a sail-like membrane and 3 rapidly moving, whip-like flagellae on its cranial end (Fig 13). In fresh specimens they move actively with a jerky motion. Diagnosis is by finding the organisms in fluid freshly collected from the stomach of an aborted fetus, uterine discharges or washings of the vagina and prepuce (Fig 14). Fluid material should be centrifuged at 2000 rpm for 5 minutes. The supernatant is then removed and a drop of sediment transferred to a slide for microscopic examination for the

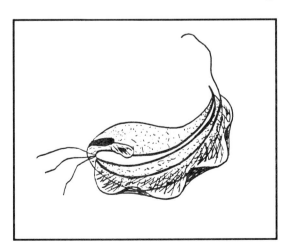

Figure 13. Diagram of *Tritrichomonas foetus*. (6000X)

Figure 14. Appearance of tritrichomonads in a preputial smear from a bull.

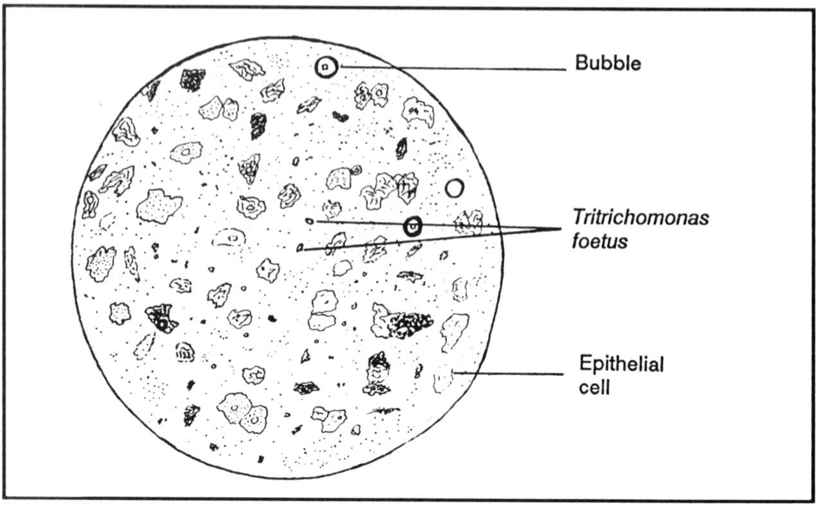

moving organisms. Several slides should be examined. For more accurate diagnosis, fluid material from the sources mentioned above can be cultured in special media. Specialized laboratories should be consulted for information on these techniques.

Parasites of Swine

Balantidium coli

Balantidium coli is an intestinal protozoan of swine. Trophozoites are usually seen in diarrheic feces. A cyst form may be seen in normal feces. The trophozoite is 50-150 μ long, with rows of cilia (short, hair-like structures) covering its surface (Fig 15).

Isospora suis

Isospora suis is an intestinal coccidian of swine. This parasite is usually found in the feces of young piglets. The oocysts are light yellow and nearly spherical, with a diameter of 18-24 μ (Fig 16). They may be seen containing one internal sporoblast (sphere) or, within 1-2 hours, containing 2 sporoblasts.

Ascaris suum

The roundworm, *Ascaris suum*, is a large, thick nematode measuring up to 30 cm long. It is one of the major internal

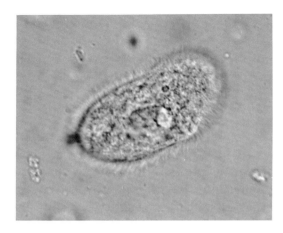

Figure 15. A trophozoite of *Balantidium coli*. (560X)

parasites of pigs throughout the world, causing huge economic losses annually. *Ascaris* typically occurs in the small intestine but can also be found in the stomach. Females can lay several hundred thousand eggs per day. Eggs remain viable in the environment for years. Infection is most prevalent in piglets under 6 months of age and causes stunted growth, unthriftiness, pot belly and diarrhea, and occasionally obstruction of the small intestine.

Ascaris larvae migrate first through the liver, causing a marked fibrosis that appears as "milk spots" on the liver surface. They then travel through the lungs, causing marked dyspnea, commonly known as "thumps" or "heaves." This condition is difficult to distinguish from viral pneumonia. Because

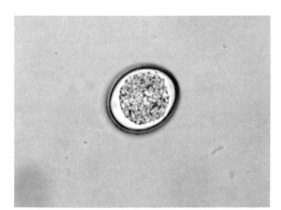

Figure 16. An oocyst of *Isospora suis*. (560X)

eggs will persist for long periods in the environment, control of roundworms is difficult.

Diagnosis: The yellow-brown eggs are slightly oval and 50-75 μ in diameter, with a thick shell covered by knobs (Fig 17). The embryo contents are undivided in fresh feces.

Trichuris suis

Trichuris suis, the swine whipworm, is the other major internal parasite of pigs. Indications are that 50-60% of herds in the midwestern United States are infected. *Trichuris* is 4-5 cm long and found embedded in the mucosa of the cecum and colon. The parasite is most often found in feeder pigs and causes dysentery about 3 weeks after infection. As with *Ascaris*, the eggs of *Trichuris* are very resistant in the environment and can survive for over one year.

Diagnosis: Trichuris suis eggs are very similar in shape and only slightly smaller than those of *Trichuris vulpis* of dogs (see Chapter 3, Fig 5).

Oesophagostomum dentatum

Oesophagostomum dentatum, the nodular worm of swine, has eggs 60-80 μ long, with a thin, smooth shell surrounding contents divided into 8-16 cells (Fig 18). The eggs of *Hyostrongylus rubidus*, a stomach worm, and *Globocephalus urosubulatus*, a

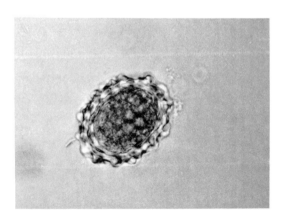

Figure 17. An egg of *Ascaris suum*. (350X)

hookworm, are similar but can be distinguished by fecal culture and larval identification.

Strongyloides ransomi

The eggs of *Strongyloides ransomi*, the intestinal thread-worm of swine, contain a formed larva surrounded by a thin smooth shell (Fig 19). They range from 45 μ to 55 μ in length.

Metastrongylus

Several species of the swine lungworm, *Metastrongylus*, cause respiratory disease in swine under 6 months of age. Signs in-

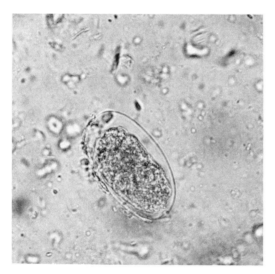

Figure 18. An egg of *Oesophagostomum dentatum*. (350X)

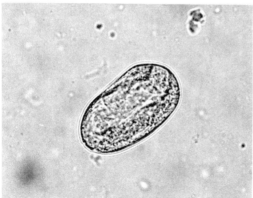

Figure 19. An egg of *Strongyloides ransomi*. (350X)

clude dyspnea, coughing, unthriftiness and death. Infection requires ingestion of the intermediate host, the earthworm.

Diagnosis: The eggs of *Metastrongylus* contain a formed larva in fresh feces but have a thicker, rougher shell than *Strongyloides* eggs (Fig 20). These eggs do not float readily in standard flotation solution and may be more easily found using sedimentation or flotation solutions with a high specific gravity (>1.250). The eggs vary from 45 μ to 63 μ in length.

Macracanthorhynchus hirudinaceus

This is the thorny-headed worm of swine. Each egg contains an embryo surrounded by 3 shell layers, with a dark-brown outer layer (Fig 21). The eggs range from 70 μ to 110 μ in length.

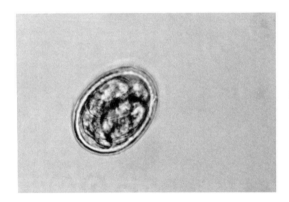

Figure 20. An egg of *Metastrongylus* sp. (350X)

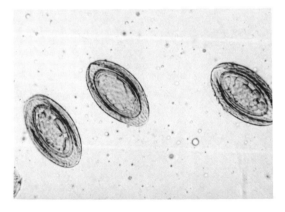

Figure 21. Eggs of *Macracanthorhynchus hirudinaceus*. (350X)

Eperythrozoon suis

Eperythrozoon suis is a rickettsial blood parasite of pigs. These organisms appear on thin blood smears as small, reddish-purple rings, 2-3 μ in diameter, on the surface of RBC or in between the cells (Fig 22). Other *Eperythrozoon* spp may occasionally be seen in the blood of ruminants.

Stephanurus dentatus

The common kidney worm of swine, *Stephanurus dentatus*, can also be found in other organs. Males are 30-45 mm long and appear a dark, blotchy color. Females are about 100 μ long, and pass eggs that flow out of the kidney in the urine. Infective larvae are ingested or can penetrate the skin. Signs of kidney worm infection include weight loss and death, with renal abscesses and hemorrhage found at necropsy.

Diagnosis: Eggs of *Stephanurus dentatus* are similar to trichostrongyle-like eggs but are larger (90-110 μ) and found

Figure 22. *Eperythrozoon suis* (arrows) in a porcine blood smear. (1400X)

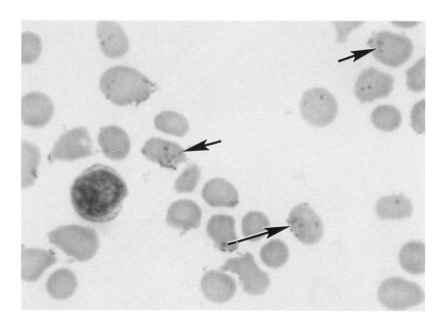

only in the urine. The contents are divided and are in the 32- to 64-cell stage (Fig 23).

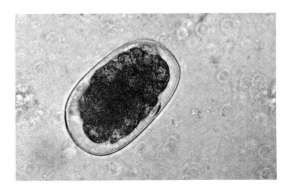

Figure 23. An egg of *Stephanurus dentatus* from swine urine sediment. (350X)

8

External Parasites of Food Animals

S.M. Gaafar

Helminths

Pelodera strongyloides

Though *Pelodera* (*Rhabditis*) *strongyloides* is usually a free-living nematode that inhabits wet and decaying bedding and moist soil, it occasionally invades bruised or eczematous skin of animals. It has been found in cutaneous tissues of cattle in various sections of the United States. Invasion by larval as well as adult stages of this parasite occurs when animals lie on wet areas contaminated with manure. The organism multiplies readily in wet bedding, as well as in skin lesions. It invades dermal tissue and may also multiply in the apocrine glands and hair follicles.

Infected skin becomes dry, scurfy, thickened, edematous and coarsely wrinkled. In severely affected areas there may be numerous pustules and loss of hair. The skin in newly affected areas is inflamed, and blood-tinged fluid may ooze from the partially depilated surface.

Diagnosis of *Pelodera* infection involves finding motile larvae and adults in scrapings or exudate from affected skin (Fig 1). Multiple skin scrapings of affected areas are required to demonstrate the small larvae. Larvae of *P strongyloides* are about 596-600 μ long.

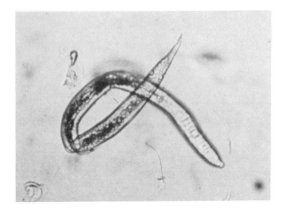

Figure 1. *Pelodera strongyloides* larva. (Courtesy of J. MacDonald, Auburn Univ)

Stephanofilaria stilesi

Several species of the filarial nematode *Stephanofilaria* infect the skin of cattle in many countries. *S stilesi* occurs in North America, Hawaii and the USSR. In the United States, this species is common in the central and western states. In some herds, 80-90% of the animals may be infested.

The lesions are usually elevated, thick, crusty areas 1-6 inches in diameter on the ventral surface of the abdomen. They may also occur on other areas of the body. The scab or crust that covers the lesions is grayish and marked with cracks and crevices. In comparatively new lesions, the crust may be red and the cracks may be moist and bloody. Older lesions usually are depilated, thick, wrinkled and cornified.

Adult worms are 3-6 mm long and about 0.1 mm in diameter. They are found in the deep dermal or subcutaneous tissues. The microfilariae, which are about 0.05 mm long, are found in the intercellular spaces, just beneath the epidermis. The presence of adults and microfilariae in the skin incites formation of cysts in which the adults are found.

Microfilariae of *S stilesi* are ingested by hornflies (*Hematobia irritans*), the intermediate host, and develop to the infective stage in about 4 weeks. Larvae are then transmitted to susceptible animals through bite wounds made by infected hornflies.

The skin lesions in cattle are characteristic. Diagnosis is by finding the adults or microfilariae in scrapings from fresh lesions. The site to be scraped is selected after removing the scabs and crusts. The scraping should be deep enough to cause slight bleeding. Adults or microfilariae may also be found in histologic sections of infected skin.

Lice

Lice are dorsoventrally flattened, wingless insects. Their bodies are divided into a head, thorax and abdomen, with 3 pairs of legs attached to the thorax. The length of adults varies from 1 mm to 5 mm, depending on the species.

There are 2 suborders of lice: Anoplura (sucking lice) and Mallophaga (biting lice). Anoplura or sucking lice are larger than biting lice. They have elongated heads, piercing mouthparts, and pincer-like claws adapted for clinging to the host's hairs (Fig 2-5). These lice are gray to red, depending on the amount of blood they have ingested. Various species of sucking lice infest all species of domestic animals, except birds and cats. Sucking lice move slowly from one area to another on the host.

Mallophaga or biting lice are usually yellow and have a large, rounded head, with mandible-like mouthparts adapted for chewing and biting (Fig 6). Several species have legs adapted for clasping, while others have legs adapted for moving rapidly. Biting lice are found on cattle, sheep, goats, horses, dogs, cats and birds.

Specific genus and species identification of each louse is difficult and is not as important clinically as differentiating the biting species from the more pathogenic sucking species.

Lice infestations are usually more serious in beef and dairy herds during cold weather than during the warm seasons. Cattle in the northern United States are infested more often with lice than are cattle in the southern regions. The tail louse (*Hematopinus pertusus*) may be found throughout the year, however, in Florida and other southern states.

Many explanations have been proposed for the abundance of lice during late fall and summer in temperate zones. The temperature of a heifer's skin in warm weather (78 F) was found to be 100 F. After exposure to the sun for 2 minutes, the skin

CHAPTER 8

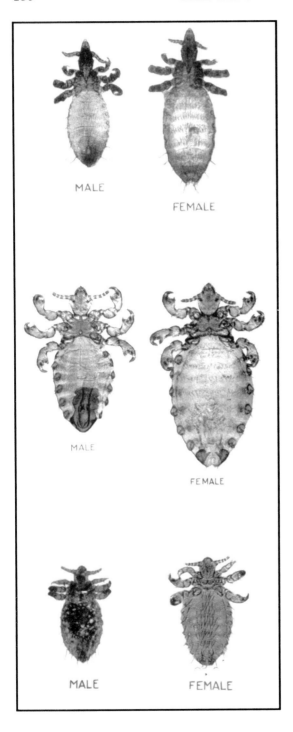

MALE

FEMALE

Figure 2. *Linognathus vituli*, the long-nose sucking louse of cattle. Note the piercing mouthparts and pincer-like claws.

MALE

FEMALE

Figure 3. *Hematopinus eurysternus*, the short-nose sucking louse of cattle. (Courtesy of D.W. Baker)

MALE

FEMALE

Figure 4. *Solenopotes capillatus*, the little blue louse of cattle. (Courtesy of D.W. Baker)

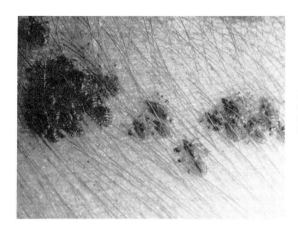

Figure 5. Sucking lice (*He-matopinus suis*) on a pig's skin. (Courtesy of L. Dunning, Univ California)

temperature rose to 125 F. Because exposure to this temperature or higher for an hour is lethal to biting lice, only lice that inhabit protected areas (inside ear flaps, brush of tail) on the host survive summer temperatures.

Transmission of lice is usually by direct contact, but adults, nymphs and eggs may also be transferred to other animals on brushes, blankets and other equipment. Lice may be transmitted easily among young, old and poorly nourished animals. There is no satisfactory explanation about why certain animals in a herd are heavily infested, while others have only a few lice. In multicolored animals, there often are fewer lice in the light areas than in the darker ones.

Ingestion of blood by sucking lice can cause anemia and may be fatal in young animals. Heavy infestations can cause the PCV

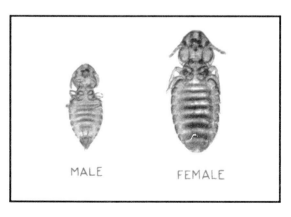

Figure 6. Biting louse, *Bovicola (Damalinia) bovis*.

MALE   FEMALE

to drop to 10-20%. Such heavily infested animals may carry as many as a million lice. They become more susceptible to other diseases and may die from stress not ordinarily injurious to uninfested animals. Poorly fed animals and in overcrowded conditions often become severely infested, anemic and unthrifty. Biting lice are much less harmful than sucking lice.

Four species of sucking lice live on the skin of cattle. *Linognathus vituli,* the long-nosed or blue louse, is about 2 mm long and common in the United States (Fig 2). *Hematopinus eurysternus,* the short-nosed cattle louse, may be 5 mm long and is probably the most common cattle louse in the United States (Fig 3). *Solenopotes capillatus,* the tuberculoid, hairy, or little blue louse, is the smallest louse of cattle, measuring 1.0-1.5 mm in length; it is not common in the United States (Fig 4). *Hematopinus pertusus,* the tail louse, is usually found in the long hair of the tail, as well as on the neck and around the eyes of cattle; it is rare in the United States.

In sheep, *Linognathus ovillus* is often found on the face, while *L pedalis* typically affects the distal legs. *Linognathus stenopsis* affects goats, and can be especially troublesome in Angoras. In pigs, *Hematopinus suis* may be found in various areas, such as the ears, axilla and neck (Fig 5).

The irritation caused by activity of biting lice during their feeding on epidermal scales, skin exudates and other skin debris and as they move over the body, causes the host to lick, scratch and rub its skin against solid objects. The resulting dermatitis gives the animal an unthrifty appearance. Because infested animals do not eat properly, they may lose weight; milk production may be reduced in dairy animals.

Bovicola (Damalinia) bovis is the common biting louse of cattle. It usually is found on the skin of the neck and withers and around the base of the tail. This louse is 1-2 mm long and pinkish yellow, with brownish bars on the body segments (Fig 6).

The biting louse of sheep, *Damalinia ovis,* is typically found on the back and head. The biting louse of goats, *D caprae,* has a similar distribution.

Life Cycle: The life cycle of lice includes 3 stages: eggs, nymphs and adults. The biology and habits of all species are similar in many respects. The eggs (nits) are white and oval, with a plug at one end (Fig 7). They are glued to the hair by the female louse and hatch in 5-14 days. The nymphs released are similar in appearance to the adults, except for their smaller size and absence of reproductive organs, genital openings, and other minor differences. After 3 nymphal instars lasting 2-3 weeks, the adults emerge. The total life cycle requries 3-4 weeks. Nymphs and adults may live no longer than 7 days if removed from their hosts. Eggs can hatch within 2-3 weeks during warm weather; they seldom hatch off the host. *Bovicola bovis* may reproduce parthenogenetically, but sucking lice require fertilization for production of hatchable eggs.

Diagnosis: Lice and nits are easily found by careful examination of suspected animals or clippings of their hair. The parasites may be overlooked, however, in animals with a thick haircoat. A hand-held magnifying lens may assist recognition of nits on the hair or adult lice crawling or clinging to the hairs (Fig 5).

Lice and eggs attached to hairs may be collected with pointed forceps and placed on a slide with mineral oil. The slide is then examined at low magnification (4X-10X objectives) (Fig 7).

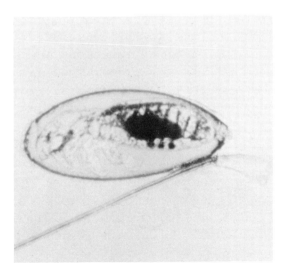

Figure 7. A louse egg (nit) attached to a hair. (Courtesy of R. Bell, Texas A&M Univ)

Flies

Many different flies attack food animals. The prevalence of any species depends on the climate, topography, and availability of water and other environmental requirements. Various species of mosquitoes and midges also attack cattle and can cause severe losses when present in large numbers. Flies cause dermatitis through their bites, transmit disease-producing organisms, and may irritate the host's ocular tissues.

Phlebotomus spp (sandflies) develop in warm, dry and sandy regions. *Simulium* spp (blackflies or buffalo gnats) multiply in rapidly running streams in mountainous areas. Both types of flies can cause severe allergic dermatitis and death. The horsefly (*Tabanus*) and the deerfly (*Chrysops*) develop near still or slowly moving water. Both are large flies whose bites are painful and may cause blood to ooze from skin punctures, through which other organisms may penetrate.

Horn Flies

The horn fly (*Hematobia irritans*) is also called the Texas fly. It is a small (3-6 mm), dark fly that lives almost exclusively on cattle throughout North America. Related species are found in other parts of the world.

When the air temperature is below 70 F, these flies often cluster around the base of the horns. In warmer areas, they may be found on the host's shoulders, back and sides, where they are least disturbed by tail switching. On hot sunny days and during rainy periods, the flies accumulate on the ventral abdomen. Dark-colored areas of the host are preferred by the flies for resting. Cattle with Brahman ancestry attract fewer hornflies.

Adult horn flies spend most of their life on cattle and leave only to deposit their eggs in fresh cow manure. The flies feed frequently, sucking blood and other fluids, and cause considerable irritation. Female flies are more aggressive than males. The energy lost in fighting the flies, together with the loss of blood, often results in reduced weight gains and milk production. Horn flies probably cause greater losses in cattle in the US than any other blood-sucking fly.

Life Cycle: Female horn flies prefer to deposit their eggs in fresh cow manure. Manure that is partially dry or crusted is not used. Groups of 5-6 eggs are deposited together, and about 20 eggs are laid at one time. A female horn fly may lay about 400 eggs during its lifetime. The eggs hatch in 16-24 hours and the larvae crawl through the manure and become fully developed in 4-8 days. These fully grown larvae migrate to the drier parts of the manure or the soil and pupate for 6-8 days. The adult fly then emerges. During hot, humid weather the life cycle may be completed in 10-14 days.

Clinical Signs: Annoyance and skin irritation are the chief effects of this fly on cattle. Because of the disturbed feeding, loss of weight and reduction in milk production may result. As much as 10-20% reduction in milk production may occur during the summer and in areas where horn flies become abundant. In heavily infested animals, severe blood loss may result in anemia.

Diagnosis: They are easily recognized by their small size, dark color, and the fact that they feed with their heads pointing down on the animal. They spend most of the time resting on their host.

Stable Flies

The stable fly (*Stomoxys calcitrans*) is also called the biting housefly or dog fly. It is slightly larger than the common housefly, from which it can be distinguished by the fact that it has a nonretractable beak or proboscis that protrudes like a bayonet. These flies occur in most parts of the world. In the United States they are common where cattle are raised, especially in the central and southeastern states. Both sexes of these flies may bite any animal. They usually attack the legs and ventral abdomen but they may also bite the pinnae.

Life Cycle: Adult females must have at least one blood meal before they deposit their eggs in wet organic material, such as straw, piles of grass, horse manure, waste silage, and other decaying matter. Each female lays about 600 eggs, singly or in clumps. The eggs, which are elongate and creamy white, hatch in 1-3 days, depending on weather conditions. The larvae feed on organic matter and become fully grown in 2-3 weeks, after which they pupate. After 6-10 days of optimum humidity and temperature, adults develop from the pupae. The life cycle may be completed in 3-5 weeks; adults may live for 20-70 days.

Clinical Signs: Though horses are the preferred host, cattle are also attacked. The fly usually lands on the host with its head pointed upward, and it does not move as much as the housefly. Both male and female stable flies inflict a painful bite that punctures the skin. The wound may bleed freely. Stable flies stay on the animal for only a short period, during which they obtain a blood meal. Though the fly is usually found outdoors, it enters barns in late fall and during rainy weather.

Stable flies have been incriminated in the transmission of anthrax in cattle and infectious anemia in horses. It is also the intermediate host for the large stomach worm, *Habronema majus*, of horses. Continued attacks on dairy cattle by large numbers of stable flies can reduce milk production. Beef cattle may refuse to graze during the daytime when attacked by these flies and, as a result, do not gain the usual amount of weight.

Face Flies

Face flies, *Musca autumnalis*, are so called because they cluster around the eyes and muzzle of livestock. They may also feed on the withers, neck, brisket and sides. These flies feed mostly on saliva, tears and mucus. They also like blood, but are unable to pierce the skin with their mouthparts, which are more suited for imbibing. They have been observed to follow blood-sucking flies, disturb them during their feeding, and then ingest the blood and body fluids on the host's skin. Face flies are found on animals that are outdoors; they usually do not follow animals into barns.

Face flies are morphologically similar to houseflies and can be differentiated through only minor differences in eye position and color of the abdomen.

Life Cycle: In general, the life cycle of face flies is similar to that of houseflies. Females lay their eggs just below the surface of fresh cow manure. The eggs are creamy white, banana-shaped, and about 1 mm long. At temperatures between 15 and 40 C, the eggs hatch in 6-12 hours. Hatched larvae feed on organic material, become fully developed within a few days to 3 weeks, and then pupate. Neither the eggs nor larvae can resist dryness. The pupal stage lasts 4-10 days, after which adult flies emerge. Under optimum conditions, a new generation of flies may be produced every 3 weeks. During the winter, they hibernate as adults in heated buildings and barns.

Clinical Signs: Face flies cause their hosts considerable annoyance despite the fact that they do not suck blood. The irritation around the host's eyes stimulates the flow of tears and attracts more flies. The continuous annoyance caused by the activity of face flies interferes with the host's productivity. Though face flies have not been directly incriminated in transmission or production of infectious keratoconjunctivitis (pinkeye), their anatomy and habits lead many veterinarians to think that they are involved.

Black Flies

Black flies (*Simulium* spp) are vicious biters that attack all species of livestock. They move in swarms, inflicting painful bites and sucking the host's blood. The ears, neck, head and ventral part of the body are common sites of bites.

Life Cycle: Females lay their eggs at the edge of swiftly flowing streams, as well as along spillways and drainage ditches. After hatching, larvae attach themselves to objects in the water. After pupation, adults can fly up to 10 miles from their hatching site. They are especially active in the morning and evening.

Diagnosis: Black flies can be recognized by their characteristic humped back and transparent wings (see Chapter 6, Fig 11).

Culicoides Gnats

Also known as "no-see-ums," *Culicoides* gnats are very tiny (1-3 mm long). They are similar to black flies in that they inflict painful bites and suck the blood of their hosts. They are active at dusk and dawn, especially during the warmer months. They tend to feed on the ventral or the dorsal area of the host, depending on the species of gnat involved.

Life Cycle: Like black flies, *Culicoides* females also lay their eggs in water, though typically in ponds, drinking troughs and other still water. Their life cycle is similar to that of black flies.

Diagnosis: In contrast to the clear wings of black flies, the wings of *Culicoides* gnats are mottled (see Chapter 6, Fig 10).

Screwworm Flies

Only one fly (*Callitroga hominovorax*) in North America is a primary invader of wounds, but there are a number of secondary and some accidental invaders. The screwworm fly is the most important fly that attacks livestock in southwestern and southern United States. It also occurs in Mexico and Central and South America. The fly may occasionally be found as far north as Kansas, but it survives the winter only in climates similar to those of southern Texas, Arizona, New Mexico and California. Several investigators believe that the fly overwinters in Mexico, close to the United States border.

The adults are greenish-blue, with a reddish-orange head and eyes, and are 8-15 mm long. The larvae can be identified through the characteristics of their caudal spiracles, pigmentation of the tracheal tubes, and other morphologic features.

Life Cycle: Female flies are attracted to fresh wounds on warm-blooded animals, where they lay batches of 15-500 eggs in a shingle-like pattern at the edge of the wounds. Several thousand eggs are laid by a female during her lifetime. The eggs are cream-colored and elongated, and hatch within 24 hours. Larvae enter the wound, where they feed for 4-7 days before they become fully grown, reaching 15 mm in length. When fully grown, the larvae drop to the ground and pupate for about a week, after which adult flies emerge.

The life cycle may be as short as 3 weeks, or up to 4 months. Larvae develop only in tissues of living animals. The ambient temperature must be above 49 F (9 C) for completion of the life cycle, especially for emergence of the adult from the pupal case.

Clinical Signs: Wounds resulting from dehorning, castration, branding, tick and fly bites, and other trauma are susceptible to invasion by screwworm fly larvae. The perineal area of a cow that has recently calved and the navel of newborn calves may also be invaded. The larvae secrete liquefying enzymes and penetrate intact tissues. During this activity they may cause hemorrhage. Infested animals may refuse to eat and some may die due to malnutrition, hemorrhage and secondary infection. Infested animals are usually depressed and often isolate themselves from the herd and rest in a shaded area.

Diagnosis: Screwworm fly infestations are more common during rainy, humid and hot weather. Before the campaign to eradicate screwworm flies in 1959, more than 40,000 infestations were reported annually in Florida and adjacent states. Identification of a primary screwworm infestation is not difficult because the larvae grow rapidly and are easily seen.

Other Fleshflies and Blowflies

These flies include species of Diptera that "blow" or deposit their eggs or larvae near or in malodorous wounds on living animals or on carcasses, excrement, garbage, or similar food sources for maggots. They include the secondary screwworm fly (*Cochliomyia macellaria*), the wool maggot of sheep (*Phormia regina*), the green bottle fly (*Lucilia caesar*), the blue bottle fly (*Calliphora erythrocephala*), the fleshfly (*Sarcophaga hemorrhoidalis*), and the housefly (*Musca domestica*).

Life Cycle: Though these flies vary considerably in their morphologic characteristics, they have similar life cycles. Their eggs or larvae are deposited in wounds of living animals or in carcasses. The pupal cases are brownish, are found on the ground, and exist for 1-2 weeks. Adults are usually found around animals and in areas with abundant decaying material. They are less pathogenic than primary screwworm flies (*Callitroga hominovorax*). Because larvae of these flies feed on necrotic tissue, wounds heal quickly following their removal.

Cattle Grubs

Cattle grubs are larvae of the flies *Hypoderma bovis* and *H lineatum*. They are also called warbles, heel flies or bomb flies. Grubs are most often found in cattle, occasionally in horses, and rarely in people. The adult flies are 13-15 mm long. Their bodies are covered with dense hair, the pattern and coloring of which differentiate the 2 species. They have rudimentary nonfunctional mouthparts and live about one week. During warm humid days, the flies are active and annoy cattle. *Hypoderma lineatum* is widely distributed throughout the US but is more common in the southern and southwestern regions. *H bovis* is usually found in the northern states.

Life Cycle: One generation of *H bovis* is usually completed annually. For *H lineatum,* the life cycle may be less than one year in some locations. Adult flies of *H bovis* are common during midsummer and those of *H lineatum* may also be active in the spring or fall. Otherwise the life cycles of the flies are similar (Fig 8). The adult fertilized female lays her eggs on hair of the legs and abdomen of cattle. The eggs are white and 1 mm long; those of *H lineatum* are glued in rows along the hair shafts and those of *H bovis* are deposited singly. Within 2-6 days, larvae hatch and burrow into the skin and subcutaneous tissues. The larvae then migrate to the abdominal cavity and reach the site for their further development in 4-6 weeks. Larvae of *H lineatum* develop in the submucosa of the esophagus; those of *H bovis* may also enter the spinal canal. They remain in these locations

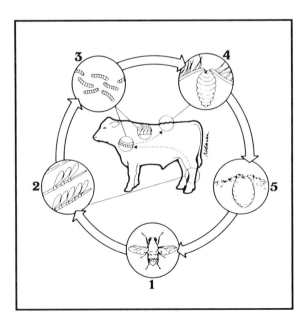

Figure 8. Life cycle of *Hypoderma bovis* and *H lineatum*. 1. mature fly, 2. eggs attached to hair, 3. larvae in esophagus and spinal canal, 4. larva on back of host, 5. pupa beneath surface of ground.

for 8-18 weeks and become about 15 mm long. The larvae then migrate to subcutaneous tissues of the back, where they bore a hole in the skin and continue to develop for 5-8 weeks. A full-grown larva is about 10 x 30 mm and dark brown (Fig 9). In the northern United States, this stage is usually reached during late winter and spring. The larvae then crawl from the breathing hole and drop to the ground, where they burrow and pupate just beneath the surface of the soil. Adult flies emerge from pupae in 1-3 months, depending on the environmental conditions.

Clinical Signs: The buzzing of the bumblebee-like flies frightens cattle. In their attempts to escape, the animals run and try to hide in shaded areas or in water. They thus may lose weight and produce less milk.

Larvae of *H bovis* in the spinal canal of cattle may cause posterior paralysis. Larvae of *H lineatum* in the esophageal wall are not pathogenic, except when they are killed with organophosphate compounds during the fall season. Esophagitis, bloat, severe shock and partial paralysis of the hind limbs have been observed following these treatments. Severe shock and death have been observed when larvae in the host's back have been crushed.

The most common lesions caused by cattle grubs are subcutaneous nodules and holes in the skin over the back. Extension of the nodule or development of an abscess can result in severe

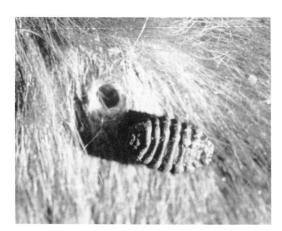

Figure 9. *Hypoderma* larva beside its breathing hole on the back of a cow. (Courtesy of L. Dunning, Univ California)

cellulitis and subsequent damage to the skin. The resultant economic loss is significant.

Keds

Keds (*Melophagus ovinus*) are dorsoventrally flattened, wingless, blood-sucking insects that resemble lice or wingless flies (Fig 10). The bites of keds cause pruritus over much of the body, damaging and staining the wool of sheep and mohair of goats. They are most numerous in the cold temperatures of fall and winter, and decline in numbers as temperatures warm in the spring and summer.

Life Cycle: Keds spend their entire 5- to 6-week life on the host. Pupae are attached to the wool or hair and mature to adults.

Diagnosis: Close inspection of the skin and wool reveals the 4- to 7-mm-long insects (Fig 10).

Ticks

These arthropods of the class Arachnida comprise several hundred species distributed throughout the world. They are

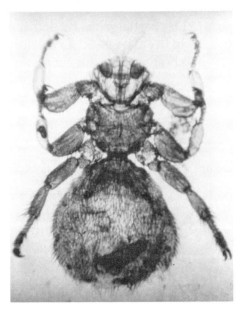

Figure 10. *Melophagus ovinus*, the sheep ked.

more common in tropical and subtropical areas, but are also found in cold climates. There are more than 40 species of ticks in the United States. All ticks must infest domestic or wild animals or birds during at least one stage of their life cycle. The fertilized female tick leaves the host to lay her eggs. Many ticks also leave their hosts during molting.

Ticks are serious pests of cattle because of the damage caused by their bites and blood-sucking. They are also capable of transmitting a number of pathogenic organisms among animals and from animals to people. The transmission of such organisms may be passive or the tick may be a necessary intermediate host.

Besides the transmission of pathogenic organisms and loss of blood caused by ticks, the salivary secretions of female ticks of some species are toxic and may cause paralysis in animals. These species include the Rocky Mountain spotted fever tick (*Dermacentor andersoni*), the Pacific Coast tick (*D occidentalis*), the paralysis tick of Australia (*Ixodes holocyclus*) and the wood tick (*D variabilis*).

Ticks are medium-sized arachnids with leathery bodies that are compressed dorsoventrally; the females are capable, how-

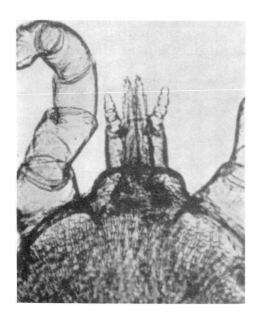

Figure 11. Mouthparts of an *Otobius megnini* nymph.

ever, of expanding their abdomen extensively when ingesting blood. The tick's head (capitulum) has cutting organs (chelicerae), a penetrating sucking organ (hypostome), and 4 appendages (2 chelicerae and 2 pedipalps) that act as sensors and supports when the tick is fastened to the host's body (Fig 11). The body of the tick may be covered partly or entirely by a hard chitinous plate, the scutum. The mouthparts may be concealed under the body or may extend from the cranial edge. Most ticks are reddish or mahogany brown, but some species have distinctive ornate color patterns on the scutum. The distal tarsal joints of the legs are armed with strong claws.

There are 2 families of ticks: Argasidae (soft ticks) and Ixodidae (hard ticks). Soft ticks have no scutum, and the mouthparts of their adults cannot be seen from the dorsal aspect.

Hard ticks are so called because they have a hard scutum that covers most of the male's dorsum and a third or less of the female's dorsum, depending on her degree of engorgement. Males are much smaller than females.

Specific identification of ticks is difficult and should be done by a specialist. Generally, however, ticks are identified by the shape and length of their capitulum, shape and color of their body, and shape and markings on the scutum. The shape and structure of the stigmal plates and nature and number of spines or spurs on coxae also assist identification. Males and un-

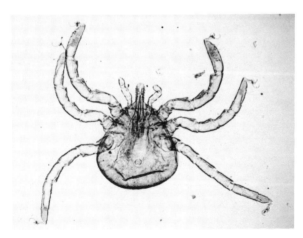

Figure 12. Tick larva.

engorged females are easier to identify than engorged females. It is extremely difficult, if not impossible, to identify larval or nymphal ticks. The common species may be identified by their size, shape, color, body markings, host, and location on the host.

Life Cycle: There are 4 major stages in the life cycle of ticks: egg, larva, nymph and adult. Following their engorgement with blood from the host, females usually leave the host and seek protected places, such as underneath leaves and branches and in cracks and crevices, to lay their eggs. Six-legged larvae (seed ticks) hatch from the eggs and proceed to feed on a host (Fig 12). The larvae molt to become nymphs, which have 8 legs and resemble the adults but do not have reproductive organs. After 1 or 2 blood meals, the nymphs become mature and molt into adults. During the larval, nymphal and adult stages, ticks may infest 1-3 different species of hosts.

Most ticks are intolerant of sunlight, dryness and excessive rainfall. They can live for as long as 2-3 years without a blood meal, but they need blood before fertilization and egg laying. Their activity is considerably reduced in cold weather. The modification of this basic life cycle among the various ticks will be discussed with each species.

Spinose Ear Tick

Otobius megnini is the spinose ear tick. Only the larvae and nymphs of this soft tick infest the ears of many domestic and wild animals. They prefer cattle, but also infest horses, sheep, goats and dogs. They are found throughout the United States, except in areas with more than 1000 mm of rainfall annually. The engorged larvae are almost spherical. The nymphs are widest in the middle of the body and are covered with prominent spines (Fig 13). Spinose ear ticks usually infest animals in sheds or corrals and seldom are found on animals in pastures.

Eggs are laid by female ticks in cracks and crevices in sheds and under feedboxes, etc. The larvae, which hatch in 3-8 weeks, can live without food for 2-4 months. When they crawl onto an animal host, they migrate to the external ear canals. Here they remain throughout the larval and nymphal stages, which may

Figure 13. *Otobius megnini* nymphs.

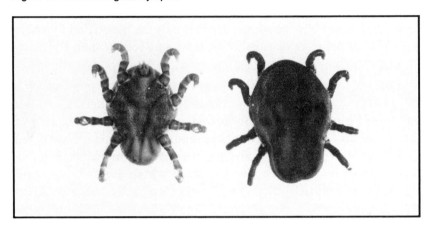

last 1-7 months. Eventually the nymphs fall to the ground and molt to become adults and lay eggs for 2-6 months.

The larvae and nymphs of spinose ear ticks live in the ear canal and deeper parts of the concha, sometimes in large numbers. They engorge themselves on their host's blood and cause constant irritation. Their feeding may also cause ulceration of the ear canal. Infested animals shake their head and tilt it to one side. In their attempt to relieve the intense itching, infested animals may bruise and lacerate the pinnae by scratching and rubbing. As the ticks increase in size, they and their excretions, together with cerumen, accumulate sufficiently in some cases to obstruct the ear canal completely. Sometimes the ticks may crawl inward as far as the eardrum. Infested animals appear dull, do not eat, and lose weight. If aural ulceration is severe, blood and exudate may attract flies that deposit their eggs there. Secondary bacterial infection may threaten the animal's life. When the lacerations and ulcerations heal and scar, the ear canals may become deformed.

Most infestations are easily detected visually. Otoscopic inspection may be necessary to diagnose mild infestations. Larval and nymphal ticks obtained from an ear canal should be identified.

Lone Star Tick

This tick, *Amblyomma americanum*, is most common in the southern states. It is also found in most of the midwestern states, as well as on the Atlantic coast. It is called the Lone Star or speckleback tick because of the white or metallic yellow spot on the apex of its scutum (Fig 14). This spot is more conspicuous on the male than on the female tick.

The Lone Star tick is found most often in the spring and summer on animals in low-lying, moist, wooded areas. It is a 3-host species and its life cycle may be completed in 3 months. There is a wide range of hosts on which this tick can survive, including domestic and wild mammals and people.

Besides the annoyance and occasional anemia that they cause, the bites of these ticks may be sites for attacks by screwworm flies. The Lone Star tick has also been incriminated in transmitting tularemia and Rocky Mountain spotted fever.

Gulf Coast Tick

Amblyomma maculatum, the Gulf Coast tick, is also called the gotch ear tick. It is a large tick often found in the ears of domestic and wild animals (Fig 15). In the United States it is common in

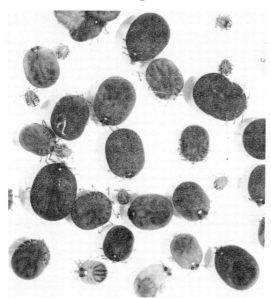

Figure 14. Lone Star ticks, *Amblyomma americanum*.

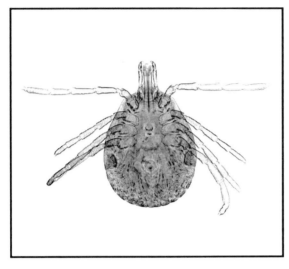

Figure 15. The Gulf Coast or gotch ear tick, *Amblyomma maculatum*.

a 100-mile-wide coastal area around the Gulf of Mexico. The tick is characterized by the silvery markings on its scutum. It is a 3-host tick and its larva may be found on birds throughout the year. The number of adults on cattle decreases during the winter and spring, and increases in summer and fall.

When in the ear canals of cattle and horses, these ticks cause severe inflammation that may cause the pinnae to droop and become deformed (gotch ear). Their bites and subsequent lacerations may become infested with screwworms.

Cattle Fever Tick

This tick (*Boophilus annulatus*) is also known as the North American tick and the Texas fever tick. It has historical fame because it was the first discovered vector of *Babesia*. The ticks as well as babesiosis have been almost completely eradicated from the United States. They occasionally are found on cattle in the most southern areas of the country.

The adults are chestnut brown and can be identified by their short mouthparts, characteristic shape of the capitulum, and shape and location of the spiracles (Fig 16).

The North American tick is a 1-host species, a characteristic that has been important in the effort to eradicate it from the

United States. It is primarily a parasite of cattle, but may occasionally be found on horses as well as deer. A closely related species, *Boophilus microplus* (the tropical cattle tick), has been eradicated from the United States, except possibly in a small area in the Florida Everglades. Strict quarantine is practiced for animals brought from other parts of the world to the United States, especially from Mexico. Whenever the tick's presence is suspected, the proper regulatory officials should be notified. The tick can then be identified by a specialist and control measures applied.

Other Ticks

Among the several other species of ticks that may infest cattle in the United States, most are 3-host ticks. The larval and nymphal forms may infest mice, rats, rabbits or other small mammals. Snakes or wild birds may serve as hosts during some stages of certain ticks' development. Among the ticks that occasionally infest cattle are: the castor bean tick (*Ixodes ricinus*) on the Pacific Coast and in Utah; the black-legged or shoulder tick (*I scapularis*) in eastern United States; and *I cookei,* which is found on cattle in California and Oregon. The American dog tick

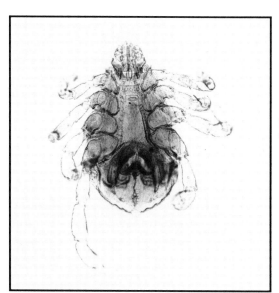

Figure 16. The North American tick, *Boophilus annulatus*.

(*Dermacentor variabilis*) and the Pacific Coast tick (*D occidentalis*) have also been found in cattle.

The winter tick or moose tick (*D albipictus*) also infests cattle. It differs from the other ticks mentioned in that it is a 1-host tick. This tick apparently attacks a wide variety of wild and domestic animals and is more prevalent during the winter months. When present in large numbers, it causes heavy losses. *D albipictus* is widely distributed throughout the northern United States, especially in elevated, wooded areas. The ticks infest their hosts from autumn until early spring. In Canada this is important because the animals are infested during the period when food is least available and their resistance is low.

Mites

Livestock may become infested with one or more species of 4 genera of mites: *Psoroptes, Sarcoptes, Chorioptes* and *Demodex.* The cutaneous diseases caused by these mites are called mange, scab, itch or barn itch. When the causal mite is identified, the condition is referred to as psoroptic mange, sarcoptic mange, chorioptic mange or demodectic mange, respectively.

Mites are minute acarids that live permanently on or in the skin of their hosts. As they feed, multiply and die, they injure the host's skin. The appearance and location of the skin lesions are usually distinctive for the mite, especially during the early stages of infestation. This is due mainly to the habits of the causal mite and to the prevailing ecologic and environmental conditions. The severity and size of lesions are determined by the number of mites, their reproductive activity, and the host's reaction.

Mites usually secrete irritative substances that react with cutaneous tissue and thus produce observable lesions. At the same time, the mites may cause irritation by burrowing in the skin. This results in scratching and self-mutilation. The skin wound may become infected with bacteria or other organisms. In demodectic mange, microabscesses and granulomas may be produced in dermal tissue. Affected animals may lose weight, be less productive, and have damaged hides.

Psoroptes

Psoroptes ovis causes common mange or body mange in cattle and sheep. *Psoroptes cuniculi* affects the ear canal of goats and sheep. Psoroptic mites are highly contagious. Though the mites that cause psoroptic mange in sheep and cattle are morphologically identical, under normal conditions they are not transmissible from one host species to the other. However, it has been demonstrated that psoroptic mites may be transmitted under experimental conditions from sheep to cattle and cause lesions in both species.

The mites are usually transmitted by direct contact or by contaminated utensils and equipment. Visible lesions can develop on newly infested animals within 15-45 days or longer. Though mites can live off their hosts for 2-3 weeks or longer under favorable conditions, they do not propagate when off their hosts. Under optimum conditions, mite eggs may remain viable for 2-4 weeks.

Psoroptic mites are small (0.5-1 mm) and oval. They have white or gray bodies, with brownish legs. The adults have 4 pairs of long legs that extend beyond the margin of the body (Fig 17). The front 2 pairs in both sexes, the third pair in males, and the fourth pair in females bear suckers with long, jointed pedicles

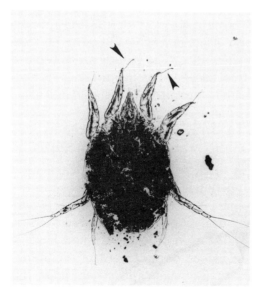

Figure 17. *Psoroptes ovis.* The arrows indicate the jointed pedicles.

(see Chapter 6, Fig 5). The mouthparts are elongated and tapering. Males are usually smaller than females.

Life Cycle: The life cycle of psoroptic mites has 5 stages: egg, larva, protonymph, deutonymph or pubescent female, and adult or ovigerous female. The adult female produces 14-24 elliptic, opaque, shiny white eggs that hatch in 1-3 days. The larvae are small, oval, soft and grayish brown, with 3 pairs of comparatively short legs. Nymphs are slightly larger than larvae and have 4 pairs of legs. Larval and nymphal stages may last 7-10 days and the complete life cycle about 10-18 days.

Clinical Signs: With their long mouthparts the mites penetrate the epidermis and suck lymph, thus causing inflammation and exudation of serum on the skin's surface. This serum mixes with skin debris and coagulates, forming a crust or scab. While feeding, mites may inject irritating substances into the host's skin that presumably provoke severe itching, resulting in additional inflammation. The mites lay their eggs under the scabs and the larvae infest the periphery of the scabby areas. The lesions thus become larger and some may become confluent, forming extensive scabby areas.

The initial lesions may be on any part of the host's body, but they are often on the shoulders, top of the neck, or around the tailhead. Other parts of the body become affected and in severe cases a large proportion of the skin is involved. Infested animals become nervous and spend a considerable amount of time scratching and mutilating their skin. The scabby areas become thick, wrinkled and fissured. Secondary bacterial or fungal infections may occur. Infested animals lose weight and some may die as a result of other diseases acquired because of stress caused by the mites. When untreated, the infestation may spread rapidly in a herd, especially among younger animals.

Diagnosis: Diagnosis is by finding the mites in typical lesions on infested animals. Though this is comparatively easy in advanced cases, the initial lesions in newly infested animals may be concealed by hair. Persistent licking, rubbing and scratching are the first indications of infestation. Infested animals become irritable and restless. Even before development of visible lesions, infested animals chew nervously and swish their tail characteristically. These early signs are usually followed by dermatitis, scab formation in the affected areas, general deterioration of health and loss of weight.

Sometimes several skin scrapings and scabs must be examined before the mites are found. If the skin is dry or the animal has been treated previously, the mites may be difficult to find. Skin scrapings should be obtained from the outer edges of lesions, where the mites are usually abundant. The scraping should be deep enough to cause slight oozing of blood.

The material obtained by scraping the skin should be mixed with a drop of mineral oil and examined microscopically (see Chapter 2). Hard scabs obtained from suspected animals may be examined by breaking them into small pieces on dark paper or on white paper with a good light. The mites appear as gray objects moving on the paper.

Chorioptes

Infestation by *Chorioptes bovis* is called chorioptic mange, leg mange or symbiotic mange. It is fairly common in dairy cattle, but is not as severe nor as fast spreading as psoroptic mange. It may occur in conjunction with another mite infestation on the same animal. The lesions are usually confined to the legs, base of the tail and escutcheon.

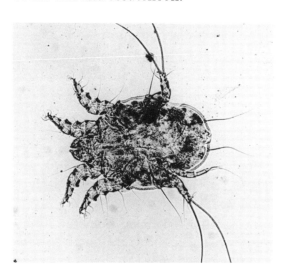

Figure 18. *Chorioptes bovis.*

The causal mites closely resemble *Psoroptes ovis*. The mouth-parts of chorioptic mites are blunt and more rounded, and the forelegs are not as thick as those of psoroptic mites (Fig 18). Short, unsegmented pedicles with broad suckers are on all 4 pairs of legs in the males, but they are absent from the third pair in females.

Life Cycle: The life cycle of chorioptic mites has 5 stages: egg, larva, protonymph, deutonymph and adult.

Clinical Signs: A large number of chorioptic mites may be present on an animal without causing observable lesions. In other animals, however, the mites stimulate formation of pap-ules and scabs on the distal limbs and over the sacrum. Lesions may then develop on other parts of the body. Though pruritus occurs, it is not as intense as in psoroptic or sarcoptic mange. Lesions are most numerous in the winter.

Diagnosis: The diagnosis is based on demonstration of the causal mites in skin scrapings. Chorioptic mites should be dif-ferentiated from psoroptic mites.

Sarcoptes

The disease caused by *Sarcoptes scabiei* is called scabies, sarcoptic acariasis or sarcoptic mange. It is an intensely pruritic disease. The mites are often difficult to demonstrate on multiple skin scrapings. For this reason, scabies is often tentatively diagnosed by the lesions and their distribution.

Among livestock, pigs are most commonly affected by scabies. Lesions caused by *Sarcoptes scabiei* var *suis* include small, red papules, alopecia and crusts, most commonly on the trunk and ears. The mites may be found in the ear wax. Similar varieties of *S scabiei* can infest people.

In cattle, scabies is a rare disease caused by *Sarcoptes scabiei* var *bovis*. The main areas affected are the head, neck and shoulders. In sheep and goats, the main area affected is the face. *Sarcoptes scabiei* var *ovis* does not affect wooled skin.

These circular mites are less than 0.5 mm in diameter. Adults have 4 pairs of short legs, of which the third and fourth pairs do not project beyond the margin of the body (Fig 19).

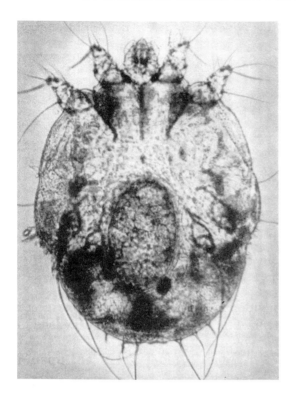

Figure 19. Female sarcoptic mange mite. (Courtesy of D.W. Baker)

Life Cycle: Female mites penetrate the keratinized layers of the skin and burrow tunnels in which they lay their eggs. About 40-50 eggs may be laid in a tunnel within 10-15 days; the female then dies. Larvae emerge from the eggs in 3-10 days and leave the tunnel to wander on the skin surface. They molt to the nymphal stage in minute pockets in the epidermis. Nymphs become adults in 12-17 days.

Clinical Signs: When they pierce the skin and feed on epidermal tissue and lymph, they cause severe irritation. The mites also may secrete substances that aggravate the irritation and cause intense pruritus. The resulting exudates coagulate on the skin and form crusts. The thickened skin becomes wrinkled, fissured, denuded and stiff. In advanced cases, infested animals scratch and bite themselves constantly and become emaciated. Some die if not treated properly. Skin over the neck and sacrum is most commonly affected, but lesions may develop anywhere on the body.

Diagnosis: The history and clinical signs usually prompt a preliminary diagnosis of mange. Specific identification of sarcoptic mites from infested animals is required for positive diagnosis. Because most of the mites are in tunnels in the epidermal tissue rather than on the surface of the skin, the deeper layers of skin must be examined. The sampled area should be scraped until blood oozes from the tissues. Several scrapings should be taken from different areas of a lesion. Scrapings from the bottom of a fold of skin will more likely contain mites.

Demodex

Infestation with these mites is known as demodectic mange, follicular mange or demodicosis. Demodectic mites live in the hair follicles of many species of domestic animals but rarely cause clinical disease. Of these, goats and cattle are most commonly affected, but then only rarely.

In goats, *Demodex caprae* occurs in small papular or nodular lesions on the shoulders, trunk and lateral aspect of the neck. In cattle, *Demodex bovis* causes large nodules (abscesses) on the shoulders, trunk and lateral aspect of the neck. The caseous (cheesy) material in these nodules should be smeared on a slide with mineral oil, covered with a coverslip, and examined for mites.

In pigs, *Demodex phylloides* rarely causes nodules on the face, abdomen and ventral neck, as well as pustules. In sheep, *Demodex ovis* rarely causes pustules and crusting around the coronet, nose, ear tips and periorbital areas.

Life Cycle: There are 5 stages in the life cycle; egg, larva, protonymph, deutonymph and adult, all of which may be found in a cutaneous nodule. The duration of various stages of these mites is not well known.

Diagnosis: Demodectic mites may be found on skin scrapings or in smears exudate from nodules. Adult *Demodex* mites are elongated, with short, stubby legs (Fig 20). Adults and nymphs have 8 legs, and larvae have 6 legs. Adults are about 250 μ long; nymphs and larvae are smaller.

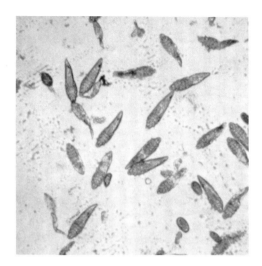

Figure 20. Demodectic mites are elongated and have stubby legs. (Courtesy of D.W. Baker)

Trombicula

Only the larvae of trombiculid mites (chiggers) are parasitic on animals and people. The nymphs and adults are free living. The larvae are most common in the late summer and early fall, and are transmitted by direct contact with foilage in fields and heavy underbrush.

The most common trombiculid mite affecting animals and people is *Trombicula alfreddugesi* (North American chigger). Of food animals, sheep are most commonly affected. Lesions consist of an erythematous, often pruritic papular rash on the ventrum, face, feet and legs.

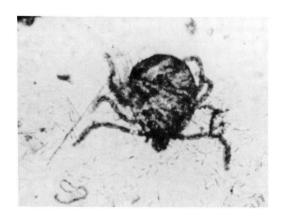

Figure 21. *Trombicula* larva.

The larvae remain attached to the skin only for several hours. Consequently, the disease may be difficult to diagnose, as the pruritus persists after the larvae have fallen off. However, scraping an orange dot on the skin may yield a 6-legged larva. Trombiculid larvae are about 450 μ long and vary in color from yellowish to red (Fig 21).

9

Parasites of Rabbits and Rodents

D.A. Shaffer and J.E. Wagner

The spectrum of parasites commonly encountered in rodents and rabbits is not much different from that found in dogs and cats seen in routine veterinary practice. Fleas, mites, round-worms and tapeworms, to name a few, can be easily detected by the veterinary technician. Identifying the species (speciation) of the parasites may be more difficult. Speciation of rodent or rabbit parasites may be critical in determining relative pathogenicity, zoonotic potential, and source of disease in cases of animals intended for resale as pets, for food or for use in research. Clients raising animals for sale as pets often keep several species of animals. These animals are likely to be housed in the same area, and cared for by a single person. The owner is often not aware of the disinfection, sanitation and isolation methods necessary to prevent cross-species infections, including zoonoses.

Most of the parasites to be discussed are relatively nonpathogenic if found in small numbers. Often, identification of a heretofore undetected parasite species in a pet animal or colony of animals is of major significance. It implies recent direct or indirect contact with other infected animals and raises the possibility of concurrent introduction of other, more pathogenic

The authors thank Dr. Craig Franklin, Dr. Susan Gibson and Dr. Judy Davis for photographic contributions, Ms. Donna Dare for typing the manuscript, Howard Wilson for taking photographs and printing illustrations, Doug Wagner for drawings, and the entire University of Missouri, Research Animal Diagnostic and Investigative Laboratory staff and faculty for their contributions to the slide and specimen collection.

parasitic, bacterial or viral agents. Even if no new animal addition can be substantiated, access by wild rodents should be suspected. Also, the ectoparasites of wild animals may be vectors of agents of some of the more pathogenic rodent and rabbit diseases. Other pets in the household should be addressed during history taking as other species of animals may be necessary hosts or vectors in some of the more complex parasite life cycles (*eg*, cestodes), or may be a source of less species-specific parasites (*eg*, fleas).

Antemortem Examination for External Parasites

Antemortem (before death) examination of rodents and rabbits for ectoparasites can be accomplished with any of four commonly used methods: hair or fur pulling, skin scraping, ear swabbing, and gross visual examination.

Hair or Fur Pulling

Hair or fur should be pulled from the section of the body appropriate for the parasite in question. These areas will be discussed later with each species of animal. The hair or fur can be plucked with forceps, placed in a Petri dish and examined under a dissecting microscope for fur mites or lice. If a parasite is found, it can usually be removed with a metal probe that has been dipped in mineral oil, and then placed in a drop of mineral oil on a slide, and coverslipped. The parasite in question can then be identified by viewing under a dissecting microscope at medium magnification. An alternative to plucking fur with forceps is to press the sticky side of cellophane tape firmly against the area of the body most likely to have pelage-inhabiting parasites. The tape is placed sticky side down in mineral oil on a slide and examined at low and medium magnification to identify parasites and ova.

Skin Scrapings

Some species of ectoparasites cannot be detected by pulling fur. Rodents and rabbits, like dogs and cats, may harbor burrowing mites, such as *Demodex* and *Sarcoptes*. As in other species

of animals, skin scrapings are appropriate for detecting demodectic and sarcoptic mange mites. Scrapings should be taken
from an appropriate area of the body, and preferably at the edge
of a lesion. Scrapings can be placed in 1-2 drops of mineral oil
on a slide and examined at low magnification. Medium power
may be necessary for speciation of the mite.

Ear Swabbing

Rabbits commonly have ear mange mites, *Psoroptes cuniculi*.
These mites can be detected by swabbing the ear canal with a
cotton-tipped applicator soaked in mineral oil or by swabbing
any brown crusty material seen on the pinnae. The applicator
should then be rolled across a clean slide, which is examined with
the microscope.

Gross Visual Examination

Antemortem ectoparasite detection can also be done with the
unaided eye. Fleas, ticks, lice and some mites can often be seen
during a careful gross visual examination of the animal.

Antemortem Examination
for Internal Parasites

Antemortem detection of rodent and rabbit endoparasites in
the veterinary clinic is usually limited to the cellophane tape
test, fecal flotation, and direct fecal smear.

Cellophane Tape Test

The cellophane tape test may be used to detect pinworm ova
of mice, rats, gerbils and hamsters. Tape tests are generally of
no diagnostic value in guinea pigs or rabbits. The tape test in
rodents is done similarly to the tape test used to detect human
or equine pinworm (*Oxyuris equi*) ova. The thumb is used on the
nonsticky side of the tape to press the sticky side of the tape
firmly to the perianal (around the anus) area of the animal. The
tape is then placed, sticky side down, on a clean slide and viewed
with the microscope at low or medium magnification. More
experienced technicians will be more comfortable using low
magnification; however, inexperienced technicians will proba-

bly feel more confident about dismissing artifacts on the slide by using medium magnification to search the slide for ova (Fig 1). In addition to pinworm ova, cellophane tape may also pick up mites and lice and their nits.

Fecal Flotation

Fecal flotation can be used to detect a variety of parasites of rodents and rabbits, including pinworm, roundworm and tapeworm ova, as well as coccidia and other protozoa. Fecal flotations may be done similarly to fecal flotations for other species of animals. Fresh feces are preferred and, in the case of rodents, are often conveniently deposited while the animal is in the clinic. It is usually necessary to request that rabbit owners bring fresh rabbit fecal specimens with them from the rabbit's cage pan. The fecal material should be crushed and mixed well in a small amount of saline or flotation solution. It may be necessary to allow the feces to soften in a small amount of saline beforehand.

Figure 1. A cellophane tape impression viewed at low (left) and medium (right) magnifications. This impression shows *Syphacia muris* eggs. Arrow points to the same egg at each magnification. The smaller object to the right of the egg is an artifact.

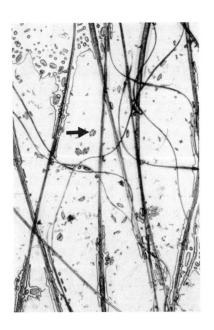 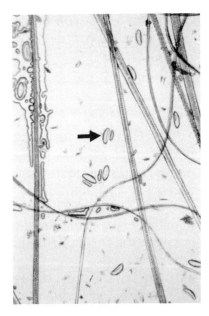

If a filter apparatus is not used in the flotation, the fecal mixture may be poured through a small funnel lined with cheesecloth or gauze to filter out large debris and allow the ova to remain in the flotation solution. The flotation solution and remaining fecal material should then be used to fill and form a meniscus on a narrow-mouthed container, such as a test tube or commercial flotation device. A coverslip is then placed on the meniscus. Maximum recovery of parasitic forms is enhanced by allowing as much as 20 minutes for flotation.

Direct Fecal Smear

The direct smear is most useful in detection of protozoal forms. Feces should first be softened with saline. Then, with a wood applicator stick, a small amount of the fecal-saline mixture can be transferred to a drop of sterile saline on a slide, gently mixed to form a thin translucent smear and coverslipped. The slide should be examined at medium and high-dry magnifications for coccidia, other sporozoa and motile protozoa.

If coccidia are found in the feces of a rabbit, fresh comminuted feces should be placed in a 2% potassium dichromate solution. This enhances sporulation of the coccidia. After sporulation, speciation of the coccidia may be possible, and the presence or absence of the more pathogenic coccidia can be determined.

Postmortem Examination
for External Parasites

Methods used for postmortem (after death) ectoparasite examination are nearly identical to those used for antemortem examination, with the addition of histopathologic examination of the skin for burrowing mites. In place of fur pulling, a portion of the dead animal's skin can be removed and placed in a dry, clean Petri dish. The fur can be examined under a dissecting microscope for mites and lice that tend to migrate toward the tips of the hair shafts as body heat dissipates.

Histologic Examination

Histologic examination of the skin can be done to detect burrowing mites. A piece of skin from the recently deceased animal should be placed in 10% buffered formalin for 24 hours. The formalin:tissue volume should be 10:1 or higher. Skin should be removed from a lesion or the appropriate area of the body for the particular mite in question. The skin specimen must be embedded in paraffin, sectioned and stained. The resulting slide can be examined for burrowing mites.

Postmortem Examination for Internal Parasites

Methods of postmortem endoparasite examination are similar to those used for antemortem examination. As with antemortem examinations, the cellophane tape test for rodents, fecal flotation, and the direct smear are appropriate. After death, direct smears may be taken directly from tissues or organs and the areas of gut most likely to harbor certain parasites, such as the duodenum for *Spironucleus muris* and *Giardia* spp or the cecum for many of the flagellates. In addition to these, portions of the cecum and colon can be placed in a Petri dish in saline (Fig 2). Adult pinworms move into the saline and can be seen grossly. The cecum and colon can be opened and the contents examined under a dissecting microscope for adult worms. The worms can be retrieved with a pipette and placed on a slide in a

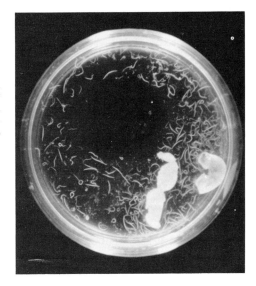

Figure 2. A 2-inch Petri dish containing saline and proximal loops of colon from 3 mice. The white hair-like objects are *Aspiculuris tetraptera* parasites that have moved into the saline from the colon sections.

drop of saline, coverslipped, and examined microscopically to identify the parasite in question.

Gross visualization of the abdominal cavity may reveal cestode larval forms (Fig 3) or pale areas in the liver suggestive of liver coccidial infection. Gross visualization of the gut lining may reveal adult helminths, such as tapeworms (Fig 4).

Figure 3. *Cysticercus fasciolaris* in mouse liver (arrow).

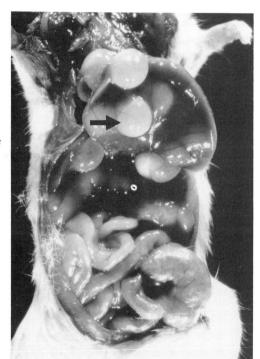

Figure 4. Intestinal lining of a mouse with numerous *Hymenolepis nana* attached.

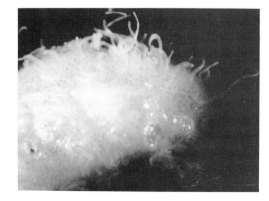

Histopathologic examination of the gut requires that the gut be gently flushed with 10% buffered formalin, fixed in formalin, processed and stained. The resulting slides can be examined microscopically for evidence of a variety of parasites.

PARASITES OF MICE
External Parasites
Lice

Polyplax serrata is the house mouse louse. It has mouthparts morphologically adapted for sucking blood from its host. Sucking lice generally are more debilitating than chewing lice. *Polyplax serrata* is 0.6-1.5 mm long. It is a slender yellow-brown to white louse with a narrow head. Like most lice, *P serrata* is large enough to be detected by careful visual inspection of the haircoat or by microscopically examining pulled hair. The adult stage of *P serrata* is most likely to be found on the forebody of the mouse. Oval nits may be seen attached near the base of the hair shafts.

Clinical signs associated with *P serrata* infestation include restlessness, scratching, anemia, unthrifty appearance and death. Dermal signs should not be immediately attributed to pediculosis (louse infestation) if a louse or nit is detected. The dermal signs may be due to other causes, such as a concurrent infestation with mites. Therefore, it is wise to thoroughly examine any animal or sample, rather than ceasing when a single parasite has been identified.

Polyplax serrata is transmitted by direct contact between mice. Because lice are species-specific, cross-contamination of other species housed in the same area, and transmission to people are not considerations. However, *P serrata* may serve as a vector for several rickettsial organisms and should therefore be handled with caution.

Fur Mites

The 3 most common fur (or pelage) mites of the mouse are *Myobia musculi*, *Myocoptes musculinus* and *Radfordia affinis*. Mice housed in close association with rats may become infested with *Radfordia ensifera*, a rat fur mite. Rodent mites have life cycles similar to those of mites of other animal species, with larval and nymphal stages. Most larval and nymphal stages have only 6 legs (Fig 5, top), while adults have 8 legs (Fig 5, center).

The first pair of legs of *M musculi* and *R affinis* are distinctly short and adapted for clasping hair. In *M musculinus*, all 4 pairs of legs are adapted for clasping hair of the host, with the first 2 pairs of legs being somewhat clublike on the ends (Fig 5, bottom). This feature distinguishes *M musculinus* from both *M musculi* and *R affinis*.

The second pair of legs of *M musculi* and *R affinis* end with clawlike features referred to as empodia. The empodia of *M musculi* are long and single (Fig 6, left), whereas *R affinis* has a shorter pair of empodia of unequal length on the second set of legs (Fig 6, right).

Adult females of *M musculi* are about 400-500 μ long and 200 μ wide. Males are similarly shaped but proportionately smaller. *Radfordia affinis* is similar in size and shape to *M musculi*. Adult females of *M musculinus* are smaller than the other fur mites of mice, measuring 300 x 130 μ. The male is 190 x 135 μ.

Mite eggs can be found attached near the base of the hairs of the host. The eggs are oval and about 200 μ long (Fig 7).

To detect fur mites on a live mouse, fur can be obtained by plucking with a forceps, or by pressing the sticky side of cellophane tape on the pelt of the mouse. The plucked fur can be placed in a drop of mineral oil on a slide and examined microscopically for mites or eggs. The cellophane tape can be placed sticky side down on a drop of mineral oil on a slide and similarly examined. Fur samples should be taken from the neck or shoulder region, as that is where the mites most commonly reside and produce lesions.

Postmortem detection of pelage-inhabiting mites of mice may be approached as in the antemortem method, or the dead mouse may be placed under a warm lamp for a few minutes. The heat attracts the mites in the pelt, causing them to move to the tips of the hairs. A hand-held magnifying glass or a dissecting microscope aids detection of the mites. The mites may then be collected on the tip of a metal probe, or similar instrument, that has been dipped in mineral oil, and placed in a drop of mineral oil on a slide, coverslipped, and examined microscopically.

The pathogenicity of mouse fur mites varies greatly with the host and the degree of infestation, much like demodectic mange of dogs. Clinical signs may be absent, or may include alopecia,

Figure 5. *Myocoptes musculinus*, a fur mite of mice. Top: Nymphal female. Note the absence of adult hind legs. Center: Adult female. Oval shape within is an egg. Bottom: Adult male with air bubble artifact.

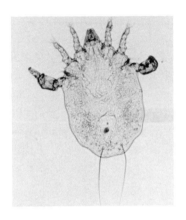

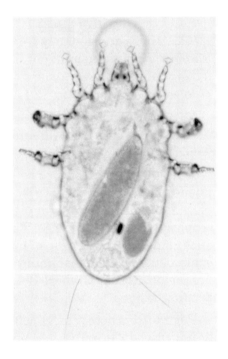

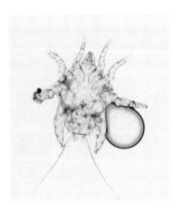

Figure 6. Left: Eight-legged nymphal form of *Myobia musculi*, showing a single, long empodial claw on the second pair of legs (arrow). The extended mouthpart is typical of the nymphal form. Right: *Radfordia affinis*, showing paired, empodial claws on the second leg pair.

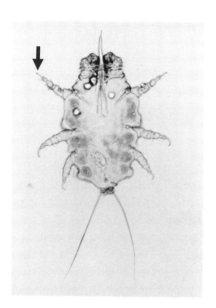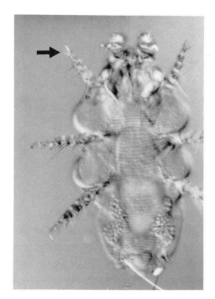

Figure 7. Nits of *Myocoptes musculinus* attached to hair shafts from a mouse.

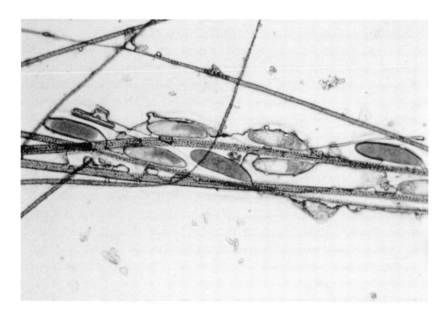

pruritus and ulceration. More severe lesions may be due to host sensitivity to the mites, in which case few, if any mites, are seen.

Transmission of all 3 mouse fur mites is by direct contact. Though mites are generally host specific, the multispecies owner should be advised that *M musculi* and *R affinis* may infest rats and guinea pigs housed in the same area with mice infested with *M musculi* and *R affinis*. The 3 mouse fur mites are not known to infest people.

Internal Parasites

Tapeworms

The mouse and rat act as intermediate hosts in the life cycle of the feline tapeworm, *Taenia taeniaeformis*. The larval form is referred to as *Cysticercus fasciolaris*. Gravid proglottids (segments) and eggs of *T taeniaeformis* are passed in the feces of the feline host. If infected feces contaminate rodent feed or bedding, the rodent may ingest embryonated eggs, which hatch in the small intestine. The embryos then migrate to the liver of the rodent, where they form a white cyst or abscesslike structure several millimeters in diameter (Fig 3). After about 30 days of development, the larvae are infective to felines that ingest the rodent liver.

It is unlikely that *C fasciolaris* will be detected antemortem unless the infection is heavy and causes the rodent to appear potbellied. Diagnosis is usually based on finding cysts in the liver of the rodent postmortem. Clients with cats and rodents should be warned of the possibility of rodent infection with this parasite. Rodent feed and bedding should be stored to preclude contamination by feline fecal material. Cats in the household should be dewormed.

Mice, rats, gerbils and hamsters are the definitive hosts of the tapeworms *Hymenolepis nana* and *Hymenolepis diminuta*. *Hymenolepis nana* and *H diminuta* are small, slender tapeworms; adult females are 25-40 x 1 mm (*H nana*), and 20-60 x 3-4 mm (*H diminuta*). Adult tapeworms reside in the small intestine of the host and are easily detected postmortem by grossly examining the contents and lining of the small intestine (Fig 4). An *H nana* adult can be differentiated from an *H diminuta* adult by the ring of hooks in the scolex of *H nana*, referred to as an armed rostellum (Fig 8). The scolex of *H diminuta* has no hooks.

Antemortem, *Hymenolepis* spp ova may be detected by fecal flotation. However, veterinary technicians should be aware that the eggs of the *Hymenolepis* spp may be shed intermittently in the feces either as individual eggs or in proglottids, which do not float. The oval egg of *H nana* measures 44-62 x 30-55 μ. The egg of *H diminuta* is more spherical and measures 62-88 x 52-81 μ. The eggs of both species contain an embryo that measures 24-30 x 16-25 μ, and that, as in all species of cestodes, contains 3 pairs of hooklets.

Clinical signs are generally not evident in light *Hymenolepis* infections. In heavy infections, diarrhea and chronic weight loss to emaciation may be observed.

Though both species are zoonotic, accurate identification of the *Hymenolepis* species is important because *H nana* is the only cestode that does not require an intermediate host. Thus, it is

Figure 8. Scolex of *Hymenolepis nana,* showing the armed rostellum (arrow).

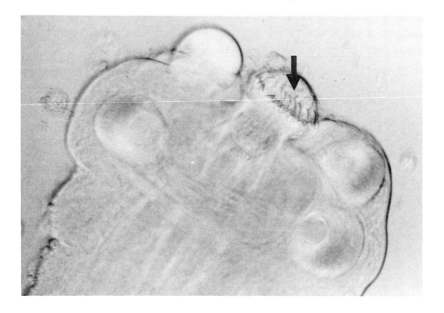

directly infective to other rodents and people. *Hymenolepis diminuta* requires an insect, such as a flea, grain beetle or cockroach, as an intermediate host to complete its life cycle. Though *H nana* can be indirectly transmitted through flour beetles or fleas as intermediate hosts, its eggs are also directly infective when ingested by any definitive host, including people. Autoinfection by *H nana* is also possible when eggs hatch in the small intestine of the host. While both *H nana* and *H diminuta* have zoonotic potential, *H nana* is considered more important because of its direct life cycle. *Hymenolepis nana* infections in people may produce vomiting, diarrhea, anorexia, loss of weight, abdominal pain, irritability, nasal and anal pruritus, and sometimes neurologic signs.

Nematodes

Oxyurids (Pinworms): Pinworms of mice include *Syphacia obvelata*, *Aspiculuris tetraptera*, and to a lesser extent, *Syphacia muris*, the common rat pinworm. Patent *Syphacia* infections can be detected ante- and postmortem with the perianal cellophane tape test described previously in this chapter. The adults of *Syphacia* reside in the cecum of the mouse until the gravid (egg-containing) female migrates the length of the colon to deposit a large bolus of eggs on the skin of the perianal region, after which the female pinworm dies.

Ova of *A tetraptera* cannot be detected with the perianal tape test. *Aspiculuris tetraptera* adults reside mainly in the proximal loop of the colon of the mouse and do not migrate to deposit ova on the perianal area, as do *Syphacia* spp. Ova of *A tetraptera* can be detected antemortem by fecal flotation and occasionally by direct smear of fecal material.

The banana-shaped ova of *S obvelata* are elongated, with pointed ends (Fig 9). They are flat on one side and convex on the other. The ova are 118-153 x 33-55 μ. *Syphacia muris* is found less frequently in mice, and in smaller numbers. The more symmetric, football-shaped ova of *S muris* are smaller (72-82 x 25-36 μ) than those of *S obvelata* and appear blunted or rounded on the ends (Fig 1). In fecal flotation preparations, the ova of *A tetraptera* have a thinner shell than the ova of the *Syphacia* and

Figure 9. Ova of *Syphacia obvelata,* the mouse cecal pinworm, as they appear on a cellophane tape preparation.

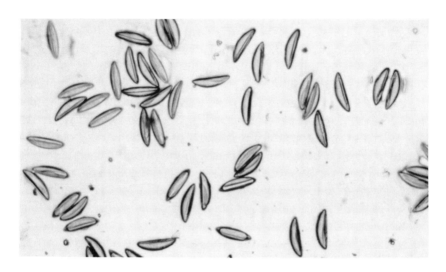

do not have a flattened side. *Aspiculuris tetraptera* ova are 89-93 x 36-42 μ, symmetrically ellipsoid, and midway in size between ova of the 2 *Syphacia* species (Fig 10).

Postmortem, pinworms of mice may be detected by placing a small piece of the cecum and the proximal loop of the colon in a Petri dish with a small amount of saline. Within a few minutes, pinworms can be seen in the saline grossly or with the aid of a

Figure 10.Ovum of *Aspiculuris tetraptera,* the mouse colon pinworm, usually seen by fecal flotation.

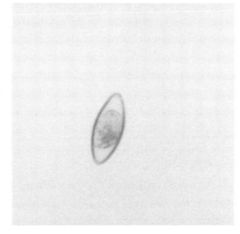

hand-held magnifying lens or a dissecting microscope (Fig 2). The adult pinworms can be retrieved with a bulb and pipette, dropped on a slide, coverslipped, and examined microscopically at low magnification. *Aspiculuris tetraptera* is usually recovered from the proximal colon and is easily distinguished from *Syphacia* spp by its oval esophageal bulb and prominent cervical alae (Fig 11, top). *Syphacia obvelata* and *S muris* are usually recovered from the cecum. *Syphacia* spp have a rounded esophageal bulb and small cervical alae (Fig 11, center). Additionally, the vulva is in the cranial one-sixth of the body of *S obvelata* females (Fig 11, bottom), whereas the vulva of *S muris* is in the cranial one-fourth of the body (Fig 11, center). Adult males of the 2 *Syphacia* species can be differentiated by the position of the 3 ventral mammelons. In males of *S obvelata*, the middle mammelon is located centrally on the length of the body (Fig 12, left). The first mammelon is at the center of the male in *S muris* (Fig 12, right). Though differentiation of the adults of the 2 *Syphacia* species may be difficult and time consuming for veterinary technicians, experienced technicians can easily differentiate the ova on the cellophane tape preparations by size and shape (Figs 1, 9).

In general, mice carry light to medium loads of pinworms without clinical signs of infection. However, heavy loads of pinworms may lead to rectal prolapse, enteritis, sticky stools and pruritus, which results in biting at the base of the tail.

Pinworms are transmitted by ingestion of the ova. The ova are hardy, resistant to environmental extremes, and light enough to aerosolize, making control rather difficult. Retrograde infection is also possible with *Syphacia* spp. For the multiple-species owner, *S obvelata* and *S muris* can be transmitted among mice, rats, hamsters and gerbils. *Aspiculuris tetraptera* has also been seen in rats. Rodent pinworms are not thought to have zoonotic potential.

Protozoa

A few flagellates may be found by direct smear or fecal flotation from the mouse. They include *Giardia muris, Spironucleus (Hexamita) muris, Tetratrichomonas microti* and *Tritrichomo-*

Figure 11. Top: Cranial end of *Aspiculuris tetraptera* female, showing the oval esophageal bulb (arrow). Center: *Syphacia muris,* showing the round esophageal bulb (arrow). Bottom: Cranial end of a *Syphacia obvelata* female. The arrow points to the vulva.

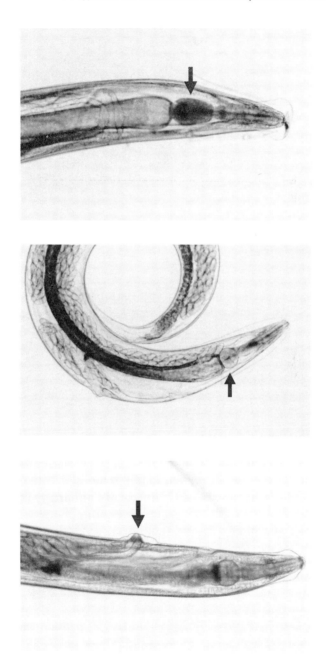

Figure 12. Top: A *Syphacia obvelata* male, showing the middle mammelon (arrow) at the center of the body. Bottom: A *Syphacia muris* male, showing the first mammelon at midbody. (arrow).

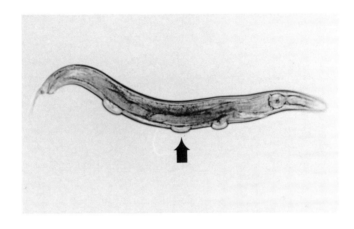

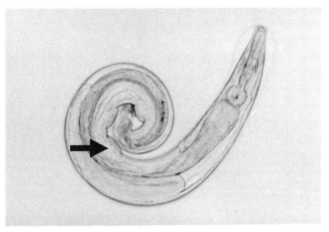

nas muris. Of these, *G muris* and *S muris* may be pathogenic. *Tetratrichomonas microti* and *T muris* are generally considered nonpathogenic.

Tritrichomonads and tetratrichomonads have 3 or 4 cranial flagella, respectively. Both genera also have a caudal flagellum. The tri- and tetratrichomonads are common in the small intestine, cecum and colon of the mouse. Animals with diarrhea, regardless of the cause, often have numerous tri- and tetratrichomonads because the diarrheic fluid medium secondarily provides an optimal habitat for tri- and tetratrichomonad multiplication. Transmission of the tri- and tetratrichomonads is by ingestion of the organisms passed in the feces. *Tetratrichomonas muris* is about 22 x 10 μ, while *T microti* is about 7 x 5 μ.

Spironucleus muris and *G muris* are the most common of mouse flagellates and have the greatest potential for pathogenicity. Both *S muris* and *G muris* occur in the proximal small intestine and can produce enteritis, particularly in young weanling mice. The location of the flagellates in the intestines is proportional to the severity of enteritis produced; the more severe the enteritis, the further back (more distally) in the intestinal tract they are found. *Giardia muris* appears similar to other *Giardia* spp. The trophozoite is piriform (teardrop in shape), with 2 nuclei at the cranial end. Eight flagella emerge in symmetric pairs from different locations cranial to caudal on the organism. *Giardia* spp may be suspected when motile forms are seen on a direct fecal smear at high-dry (100X) magnification. *Giardia* spp are identified by staining the direct fecal smear with iodine, preferably Lugol's iodine, which enhances the definition of the 2 cranial nuclei and flagella.

Transmission of *G muris* is by ingestion of cysts that have passed in the feces. *Giardia muris* has also been found in the rat and hamster; therefore, the multi-species owner should be made aware of the possibility of cross-contamination. Though other species of *Giardia* are pathogenic to people, the *Giardia* spp found in rodents and rabbits have no known zoonotic potential.

Spironucleus muris appears somewhat similar to *Giardia* spp except that the trophozoite of *S muris* is uniformly slender, as opposed to the widened cranial end of the *Giardia* spp. *Spironucleus muris* has 2 cranial nuclei. There are 3 pairs of cranial flagella, and one pair of trailing caudal flagella (Fig 13).

Sporozoa

Intestinal Coccidia: Cryptosporidium spp are coccidian parasites in the suborder Eimeriorina, which also includes *Eimeria* and *Isospora*. The Eimeriorina are enteric coccidia that use a single host in their life cycle (monoxenous).

Figure 13. *Spironucleus (Hexamita) muris* cyst (left) and trophozoites (right).

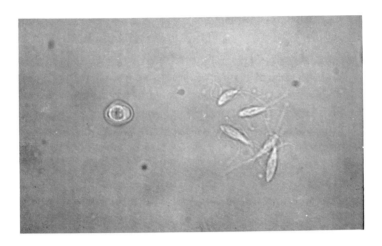

The *Cryptosporidium* spp associated with mice (*C parvum* and *C muris*) are small (3-7 μ), round to oval enteric parasites. *Cryptosporidium muris* is found in the stomach, attached to the epithelial surface or in the lumen of the gastric glands, while *C parvum*, like the other *Cryptosporidium* spp, is found in the small intestine, attached to and embedded in the tips of epithelial cells lining the intestinal villi. Concentrations of *C parvum* are highest in the ileum.

Cryptosporidium spp may be detected antemortem by the oocysts in fecal flotation preparations using light or phase-contrast microscopy. Concentration techniques, such as fecal flotation with Sheather's sugar solution, may enhance recovery of oocysts. Small oocysts (2-6 μ) may be mistaken for yeasts. A second antemortem method for detection of oocysts relies on formalin fixation of a fecal smear and subsequent staining with acid-fast or Giemsa stains.

Postmortem, *Cryptosporidium* spp can be found histologically in hematoxylin and eosin-stained intestinal sections. The organisms are attached to the surface of the epithelium of the intestinal villi.

Cryptosporidium muris and *C parvum* are thought to be relatively nonpathogenic. Clinical signs of *Cryptosporidium* infection are rare. They include lethargy, rough haircoat, failure to gain or maintain weight, and weight loss.

Transmission of *Cryptosporidium* is believed to be by the fecal-oral route. Infectious fecal material, and contaminated feed, water or bedding are possible sources of infection. Because *Cryptosporidium* may be zoonotic, care should be taken in handling suspect animals, as well as fomites from the environment of these animals.

Several coccidia infect mice, including *Eimeria falciformis*, *E ferrisi* and *E hansonorum*. *Eimeria falciformis* and *E hansonorum* affect the small intestine, while *E ferrisi* is found in the cecum. Though mixed infections can occur, little is known about the incidence and pathogenicity of *E ferrisi* and *E hansonorum*.

Eimeria falciformis is common in wild mouse populations. Oocysts are 14-26 x 11-24 μ, round to oval, smooth and colorless. There is no micropyle or residuum. Sporocysts are oval and have a residuum and a small Steida body. There are 2 sporocytes per sporocyst, and 4 sporocysts per sporulated oocyst. Oocysts of *E ferrisi* and *E hansonorum* appear similar to those of *E falciformis*, except they are smaller (16-18 μ) and more spherical. *E ferrisi* has a small Steida body on the sporocysts, while *E hansonorum* has a broad Steida body.

Oocysts of the *Eimeria* spp can be detected by fecal flotation. As in coccidial infections of other species, finding oocysts in a fecal flotation preparation does not necessarily mean that *Eimeria* spp are a primary cause of disease. Diagnosis is made by considering clinical signs, enteric lesions, and identification of the coccidia in stained tissue sections.

Clinical signs, if seen, are usually in younger animals that have developed little or no immunity, and may include diarrhea, catarrhal enteritis, anorexia, hemorrhage and epithelial sloughing of the intestine.

As with other *Eimeria* spp, transmission is by ingestion of sporulated oocysts that have been passed in the feces. Oocysts passed in the feces sporulate in about 3 days. *Eimeria* spp are host specific and so are not considered to be a zoonotic hazard.

Kidney Coccidia: Klossiella muris is a relatively nonpathogenic coccidian that occurs mainly in the kidneys of wild and laboratory mice, but has been found in different stages of its life cycle in adrenal, thyroid, brain, lung and spleen. The oocyst of *K muris* matures in the endothelial cells that line arterioles and capillaries associated with the glomeruli of the kidney. At maturation, the oocyst is 40 μ in diameter. The oocyst grows and divides to form sporoblasts, which eventually rupture the host endothelial cell and pass through the urine as sporocysts. Other mice are then infected by ingestion of sporulated sporocysts.

K muris cannot be detected antemortem. Postmortem, the kidneys may appear enlarged and have small gray necrotic areas on the surface. When histologic preparations of the kidneys are examined microscopically, most of the necrotic areas are seen at the corticomedullary junction. *K muris* infection is usually diagnosed from the gross and microscopic lesions, including finding the organism in the tissue.

Transmission of *K muris* is by ingestion of the sporulated sporocysts passed in the urine. Because wild mice can carry this parasite, strict sanitation and prevention of wild mouse access to the pet population are needed to control this parasite. *K muris* is species specific and is not considered a public health problem.

PARASITES OF RATS
External Parasites

Lice

Like *Polyplax serrata* in the mouse, the rat louse, *Polyplax spinulosa*, is a blood-sucking or Anopluran louse. *Polyplax spinulosa* is similar to *P serrata*, and like *P serrata*, has a narrow head, with mouthparts adapted for sucking blood from the rat.

Polyplax spinulosa may be detected by gross visual examination of the midbody and shoulders of the rat. Hair may be pulled from these areas and examined for adults, nymphs or nits. Nymphs resemble small pale adults. Nits can be found attached to the base of the hair shafts. Clinical signs include restlessness, scratching, anemia and debilitation. Transmission of *P spinulosa* is by direct contact. Because lice are species specific, transmission to other species or people is not a concern. *Polyplax spinulosa* is a vector responsible for spread of *Hemobartonella muris* and *Rickettsia typhi* between rats. *Rickettsia typhi* can also be transmitted to people from infected rats by rat fleas.

Blood-Sucking Mites

Ornithonyssus (Liponyssus) bacoti, commonly called the tropical rat mite, can cause severe problems in rats and mice. This mite can also affect hamsters and guinea pigs. The mite has a wide host range beyond rodents and is especially common in tropical and subtropical climates. A blood-sucking mite, *O bacoti*, is from the suborder Mesostigmata and is more closely related to the ticks than mites. This unusual mite lives most of its life off the host animal. Both females and males are blood suckers. The females are relatively large. Depending on whether or not they are blood filled, they measure up to 750 μ in length (Fig 14).

Ornithonyssus bacoti intermittently feeds on rodent blood, dropping into nests or surrounding cracks and crevices between feedings. The mite can gain access to pet animals by dropping

Figure 14. *Ornithonyssus bacoti*, the tropical rat mite.

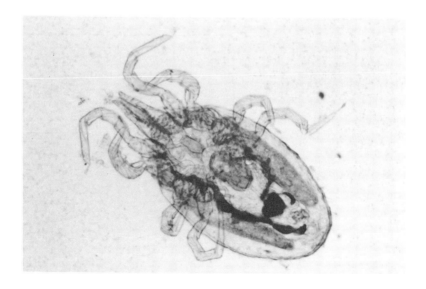

from wild or feral animals; then days later they attack a pet animal for a blood meal when the original host is no longer in the area.

Infestation with *O bacoti* is usually diagnosed by observing the blood-filled mites in bedding, nests, or cracks and crevices near pet animal cages. Animals in an *O bacoti*-infested environment may be anemic and show a marked reproductive decline. The mite can transmit rickettsial organisms, and can cause allergic dermatitis in people. In the absence of a suitable rodent host, *O bacoti* will readily attack people for a blood meal.

Burrowing Mites

Notoedres muris is also referred to as the ear mange mite of rats (Fig 15). It resembles *Sarcoptes scabiei*, with a rounded body, suckers on the first 2 pairs of legs of females, and of the first, second and fourth pairs of legs of males. Females can be distinguished from *S scabiei* females by the dorsal anal opening of *N muris*. The anal opening of *S scabiei* is terminal (Fig 16).

The mite, *N muris*, can usually be detected and diagnosed, before and after death, by collecting deep skin scrapings from the edges of suspected lesions. Lesions are usually on the unfurred parts of the body, such as the ear pinnae, tail, nose and

Figure 15. Line drawing of a *Noto-edres muris* female, showing the subterminal anal opening.

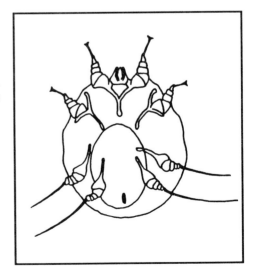

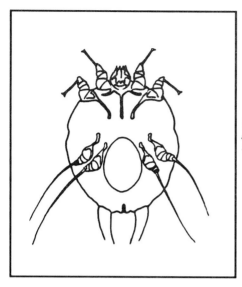

Figure 16. Line drawing of a *Sarcoptes scabiei* female, showing the terminal anal opening.

extremities. Lesions appear as crusted areas with reddened vesicles. *Notoedres muris* is fairly common in wild rodents. Transmission is by direct contact, so owners should be cautioned to keep pet rats safely away from wild rodent contact. The mite is also known to infest guinea pigs, but does not infest people.

Fur Mites

Radfordia ensifera, a fur mite of rats, is similar to *M musculi* and *R affinis* (Fig 6), which were previously discussed in the mouse ectoparasite section. *Radfordia ensifera* is distinguished from *M musculi* and *R affinis* by the empodial claws of the second pair of legs. *Myobia musculi* has a single, long empodial claw (Fig 6, left), while *R ensifera* and *R affinis* both have a pair of shorter claws. The 2 empodial claws of *R ensifera* are of equal length (Fig 17), while those of *R affinis* are of unequal length (Fig 6, right).

Antemortem or postmortem, *R ensifera* is detected using methods described for mouse fur mites. Light infestations of *R ensifera* usually cause no clinical signs while self-inflicted trauma may be seen in heavy infestations. Transmission is by direct contact. *R ensifera* is not known to infest people.

Figure 17. Second leg of *Radfordia ensifera,* showing equal length of the empodial claws (arrow).

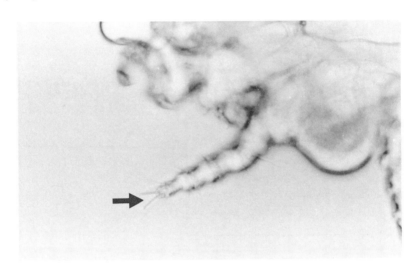

Internal Parasites

Tapeworms

Like mice, rats and other rodents can be intermediate hosts of the feline tapeworm, *Taenia taeniaeformis.* The information on this parasite in the mouse section also pertains to rats (Fig 3).

Like mice, hamsters and gerbils, rats are a definitive host for *Hymenolepis nana* (the dwarf tapeworm) and *H diminuta* (the rat tapeworm). The discussion in the mouse section also pertains to rats (Figs 4, 8).

Nematodes

Oxyurids (Pinworms): The 3 oxyurids discussed in the mouse section, *Syphacia muris, S obvelata* and *Aspiculuris tetraptera,* may infect rats. *Syphacia muris* is by far the most common of the 3 in rats, and is considered the rat pinworm (Fig 11, center; Fig 12, bottom). Methods for detection, identification, clinical signs and transmission are similar to those discussed in the mouse endoparasite section.

Threadworms: Trichosomoides crassicauda is the urinary bladder threadworm of rats. Infection with *T crassicauda* may be in 3 ways: ante- or postmortem microscopic observation of ova in the urine; gross observation of adult worms in the wall and/or lumen of the urinary bladder postmortem, and microscopic observation of the adult worms in histologic sections of the urinary bladder, ureters, or renal pelvis postmortem.

The *T crassicauda* female is a long (about 10 mm), thin worm, visible grossly in the wall of the urinary bladder of rats postmortem. The male lives in the vagina of the immature female, and then within the uterus of the adult female. Ova are about 65 x 33 μ, and doubly operculated, resembling the ova of the canine whipworm, *Trichuris vulpis*. As a comparison, the ova of *T crassicauda* are lighter in color and are slightly smaller than those of *T vulpis*.

There are few clinical signs of *T crassicauda* infection. Transmission is by the urinary-oral route. It is species specific and so is not considered a public health problem.

Protozoa

Flagellates: Though somewhat less susceptible than mice, rats may be infected with the flagellates discussed previously in the mouse section of this chapter, *Giardia muris, Spironucleus muris, Tetratrichomonas microti* and *Tritrichomonas muris*. Identification, detection, clinical signs and transmission in rats are similar to those discussed in the mouse section (Fig 13).

Coccidia

Eimeria nieschulzi is an intestinal coccidian uncommon in laboratory rats but common in wild rats. The mature oocyst of *E nieschulzi* is oval, 16-26 x 13-21 μ, with no residuum. It has a smooth or colorless wall, with no micropyle. The mature oocyst contains 4 oval sporocysts, each with a small Steida body and a residuum.

Antemortem, *E nieschulzi* may be detected by finding the oocysts in fecal flotations or direct fecal smears. However, diagnosis is usually based on identification of the organism histologically in sections of the intestinal epithelium. Clinical signs of *E nieschulzi* infection are usually seen in young rats less than several months of age. Signs include diarrhea, weakness, emaciation and possibly death. Rats become infected with *E nieschulzi* by ingestion of sporulated oocysts in feces. *Eimeria nieschulzi* is species specific and therefore is not considered a potential cross-species contaminant or zoonotic problem.

PARASITES OF HAMSTERS
External Parasites
Blood-Sucking Mites

Ornithonyssus bacoti, the tropical rat mite, can infest hamsters. Identification, detection, clinical signs, transmission and public health importance are discussed in the rat ectoparasite section (Fig 14).

Follicle-Inhabiting Mites

Demodex spp have an elongated cigar-shaped body with 4 short legs on the cranial portion. *Demodex aurati* (Fig 18) and *D criceti* (Fig 19) infest hamsters. Like other *Demodex* species, they live in hair follicles. Deep skin scrapings at the edges of lesions are necessary to detect the mites. Lesions are most often seen on the dorsum of the hamster, near the rump.

Clinical signs that may indicate demodicosis include alopecia, dry scaly skin and/or scabby dermatitis, particularly over the rump and on the back of the hamster. Demodicosis is most often seen in aged or otherwise stressed hamsters. The mite population in hamsters is usually greater in males than in females. *Demodex aurati* and *D criceti*, like *D canis*, may be present without clinical signs.

Demodicosis may be detected postmortem by histologic exam of skin sections. It is also possible to use a warm lamp to draw mites to the hair shaft tips. Transmission is by direct contact, with the primary route thought to be from mother to suckling young. *Demodex* mites of hamsters are considered species specific, with possible exception of the gerbil, and so are not likely to cross contaminate other species or pose a zoonotic problem.

Figure 18. *Demodex aurati*, a burrowing mite of hamsters.

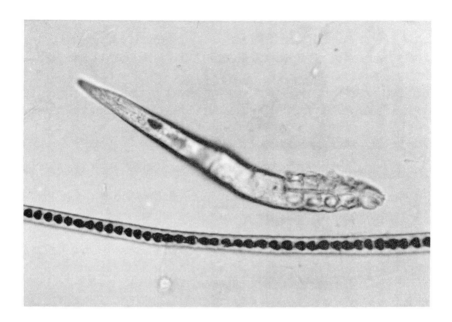

Figure 19. *Demodex criceti*, a hamster mite, distinguishable from *Demodex aurati* by its blunt body shape.

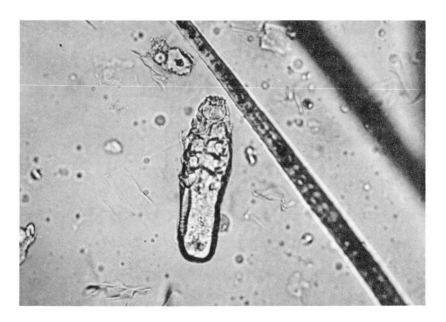

Internal Parasites

Tapeworms

Hamsters seem to be infected with zoonotic *Hymenolepis* spp tapeworms more frequently than other species of rodents. This implies that, as a species, hamsters may be more susceptible to hymenolepid infections than other pet and laboratory rodents. Identification, detection, clinical signs, transmission and public health importance of these zoonotic parasites are discussed in the mouse endoparasite section (Figs 4, 8).

Protozoa

Hamsters commonly carry numerous intestinal flagellates, that can be seen in fecal flotations or direct smear preparations, without showing clinical signs. These flagellates include *Giardia* spp, *Spironucleus muris*, *Tetratrichomonas microti* and *Tritrichomonas muris* (*criceti*). Infected hamsters may serve as a source of infection for more susceptible rodents, such as transmission of *S muris* to mice.

Identification, detection, clinical signs, transmission and public health importance of these flagellates have been discussed in the mouse endoparasite section (Fig 13).

Nematodes

Oxyurids (Pinworms): Hamsters are susceptible to infection with the mouse and rat pinworms, *Syphacia obvelata* and *S muris*, though it is unlikely they will develop clinically apparent infections. Identification, detection, clinical signs, transmission and public health importance of rodent oxyurids are discussed in the mouse endoparasite section (Figs 1, 9, 11, 12).

PARASITES OF GERBILS
External Parasites

Mites

Gerbils have been reported to carry 2 species of *Demodex* mites, *D aurati* (Fig 18) and *D criceti* (Fig 19). These are similar in size and shape to hamster demodectic mites. Demodectic mites have also been recovered from gerbils with facial dermatitis. As in other species with demodectic mange, infested animals have some other concomitant disease. Lesions are similar to those described in the hamster ectoparasite section.

Internal Parasites

Tapeworms

Gerbils are one of the definitive hosts of the dwarf tapeworm, *Hymenolepis nana*. A heavy infection can cause mucoid diarrhea and death. A more complete discussion of the identification, clinical signs, transmission and public health importance of this zoonotic parasite can be found in the mouse section (Figs 4, 8).

Nematodes

Oxyurids (Pinworms): Dentostomella translucida, the gerbil pinworm, is not reported as frequently as other rodent pinworms (*Syphacia* and *Aspiculuris tetraptera*). This may be due in part to the lack of information on its life cycle. Adult worms, male and female, have a short muscular esophagus. The vulva of the female is located just cranial to the midbody (Fig 20). Males are distinguished by a cuticular inflation just cranial to the cloaca (Fig 21). Adults are 6-31 mm long, with the female generally larger than the male, as is true of the other rodent pinworms. Ova of *D translucida* are asymmetrically oval, 120-140 x 30-60 μ (Fig 22), and resemble those of *Aspiculuris tetraptera*, which are smaller (89-93 x 36-42 μ).

Antemortem, fecal flotation may be used to detect ova of *D translucida*, but this method is unreliable due to the poorly understood life cycle (intermittent shedding of ova). Postmortem, *D translucida* may be seen in the proximal one-third of the small intestine.

Dentostomella translucida has a direct life cycle and is transmitted by ingestion of infective ova in feces of infected animals. This parasite has been found in the golden hamster as well as the gerbil. It is not considered a public health problem.

Like hamsters, gerbils are susceptible to infection with the mouse and rat pinworms, *Syphacia obvelata* and *S muris* (Figs 1, 9, 11, 12). Identification, clinical signs, transmission and

Figure 20. An adult female *Dentostomella translucida.*

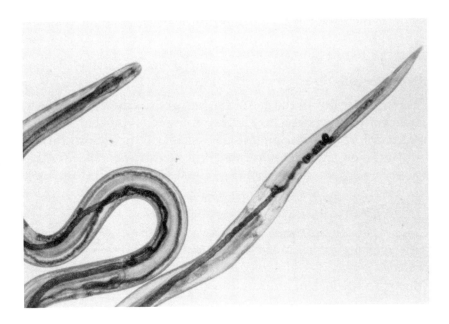

Figure 21. Cuticular inflation (arrow) on the tail of a male *Dentostomella translucida.*

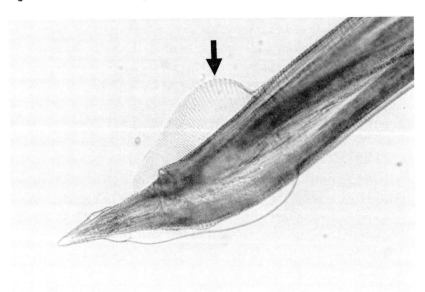

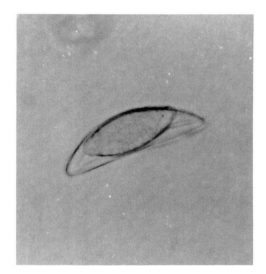

Figure 22. Egg of *Dentostomella translucida* in a fecal flotation.

possible public health importance are discussed in the mouse section.

PARASITES OF GUINEA PIGS
External Parasites

Lice

Gliricola porcelli and *Gyropus ovalis* are the lice of guinea pigs. Both belong to the order Mallophaga or chewing lice. They differ from those of the order Anoplura, or sucking lice, by their somewhat triangular head, with a strong pair of mandibles used to abrade skin and obtain cutaneous fluids. *Gliricola porcelli* and *G ovalis* belong to the family Gyropidae, distinguished by having one or no claws on the second and third pairs of legs.

Gliricola porcelli is known as the slender guinea pig louse and is 1.0-1.5 x 0.3-0.44 mm (Fig 23). *Gyropus ovalis*, as its name implies, is more oval than *G porcelli* and measures 1.0-1.2 x 0.5 mm (Fig 24). The head of *G ovalis* is much broader than that of *G porcelli*. Of the 2, *G porcelli* is more common.

Guinea pig lice can be detected antemortem by careful inspection of the haircoat, either grossly or with a hand-held magnifying glass. Postmortem, a method similar to that used to detect lice in other species of animals may be useful. That is, a piece of the pelt from the dead animal may be placed in a covered Petri dish and placed under a mild heat source, such as a small reading lamp. In a short time, as the pelt cools, the lice migrate toward the warmth and to the tips of the hairs. The lice can be easily seen grossly or with a hand-held magnifying glass.

Figure 23. *Gliricola porcelli,* the slender guinea pig louse.

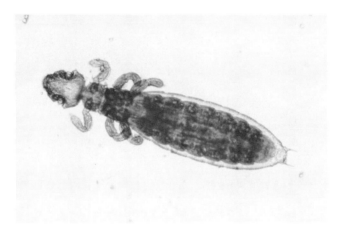

Figure 24. *Gyropus ovalis,* a less common guinea pig louse.

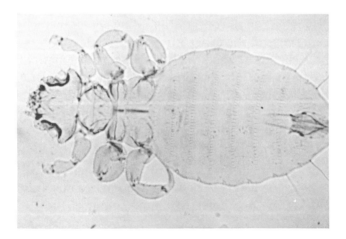

Light infestations of *G porcelli* or *G ovalis* usually cause no clinical signs. However, in heavy infestations, alopecia and scab-like areas may develop, especially in the areas caudal to the ears of the guinea pig. Excessive scratching may be noticed.

Transmission of *G porcelli* and *G ovalis* is by direct contact, with another host guinea pig or bedding or other fomites from infested guinea pigs. Like other lice, guinea pig lice are species specific and do not cross infest other species, including people.

Fur Mites

The fur mite that commonly infests guinea pigs is *Chirodiscoides caviae*. *Chirodiscoides caviae* is an elongated mite, with a triangular cranial portion that appears like the head of the mite. All legs are adapted for clasping hair. There are no empodial claws on the first 2 pairs of legs. The male is about 363 x 138 μ (Fig 25) and the female is 515 x 164 μ (Fig 26).

It is somewhat difficult to observe *C caviae* antemortem with the unaided eye. *Chirodiscoides caviae* may be detected antemortem by pulling hairs, either with forceps or by the cellophane tape method, and then examining the specimen microscopically. *Chirodiscoides caviae* is found in the pelt in the greatest numbers over the rump. Postmortem, a piece of the pelt from the rump of the dead animal may be placed in a Petri dish to cool and is examined with a hand-held magnifying glass or with a dissecting microscope for mites at the tips of the hairs.

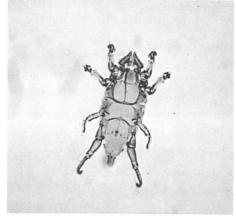

Fgure 25. *Chirodiscoides caviae* male, a fur mite of the guinea pig.

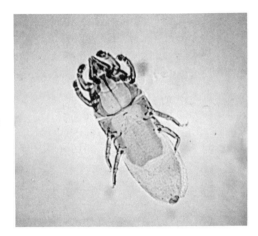

Figure 26. Female *Chirodiscoides caviae.*

Usually there are no clinical signs unless infestation is severe, when alopecia and pruritus may be seen. Though *C caviae* is not considered transmissible to people, transient infestations causing a pruritic, papular urticarial skin condition have been reported in people.

Myocoptes musculinus and *Radfordia affinis*, the fur mites of mice, are also transmissible to guinea pigs. These mites are discussed in the mouse ectoparasite section (Figs 5, 6).

Burrowing Mites

Another mite that commonly infests guinea pigs is *Trixacarus caviae* (Fig 27). *Trixacarus caviae* is a typical sarcoptid mite, with a rounded body and suckers on long, unjointed stalks on the first 2 pairs of legs of females and on the first, second and fourth pairs of legs of males.

Deep skin scraping from the edges of suspected lesions around the back, neck and shoulders is necessary to detect this mite ante- and postmortem. Lesions include dry, scaly skin, with pruritus, alopecia and dermatitis, resulting in hyperkeratosis.

Other burrowing mites that may infest guinea pigs are *Sarcoptes scabiei* (Fig 16) and *Notoedres muris* (Fig 15). *Sarcoptes scabiei* can be transmitted from rabbits to guinea pigs, where they produce scabby lesions on the nose and lips. Young guinea

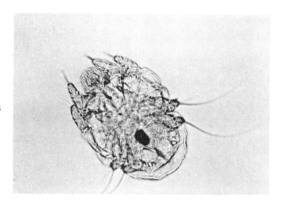

Figure 27. *Trixacarus caviae*, a sarcoptid mite of guinea pigs.

pigs are particularly susceptible and may become anorectic to the point of death if not treated. Identification, detection and transmission of *S scabiei* are more thoroughly discussed in the rabbit ectoparasite section. *Notoedres muris* is generally associated with rats but also has been reported in guinea pigs. This mite produces red crusty lesions on the face of guinea pigs. Identification, detection and transmission are discussed in the rat section.

Internal Parasites

Nematodes

Paraspidodera uncinata is generally a nonpathogenic ascarid of guinea pigs that can be found in cecal contents or on the mucosa of the cecum and colon. Adult worms are 11-28 mm x 0.3-0.4 mm. The male of *P uncinata* has a sucker and 2 spicules of equal length immediately cranial to the anus. The ova are oval, with a typical thick ascarid shell (Fig 28). Ova measure 40-50 x 30-40 μ. Antemortem, ova may be detected by fecal flotation or direct fecal smear. Occasionally, very heavy infections may cause diarrhea and weight loss.

The life cycle is direct and transmission occurs through feed and water contaminated with infective ova that have passed in the feces. *Paraspidodera uncinata* has not been found in other species of animals and is not considered a public health hazard.

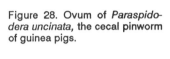

Figure 28. Ovum of *Paraspido-dera uncinata*, the cecal pinworm of guinea pigs.

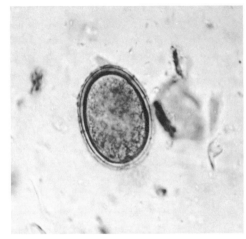

Protozoa

Amoebae: Entamoeba caviae is a relatively common non-pathogenic cecal organism in guinea pigs. It is mentioned in this chapter so that the technician can be aware to disregard it as a pathogenic organism when it is seen.

Trophozoites are the form of *E caviae* usually seen. Cysts are not commonly found except by concentration with zinc sulfate flotation. Mature cysts, when they are found, measure 11-27 μ and have 8 nuclei. The trophozoites are most often found in a direct fecal smear and measure 10.5-20.0 μ in diameter. The appearance of the trophozoites can be enhanced by staining a direct fecal smear with Lugol's iodine.

Entamoeba caviae is transmitted by ingestion of infective cyst forms that have been passed in the feces of chronic carrier guinea pigs. *Entamoeba caviae* is species specific and not considered a zoonotic threat.

Flagellates

Trophozoites of *Giardia caviae* are similar to those of *G muris* previously discussed. The body is piriform or teardrop in shape. Two nuclei lie at the cranial end and 4 pairs of flagella emerge at various points of the body. Trophozoites are 8-15 x 6.5 μ. Cysts are about the same size as the trophozoites and contain 2-4 nuclei.

Cysts or trophozoites of *G caviae* may be detected in a direct fecal smear, or possibly in a fecal flotation preparation. If fecal flotation is used, zinc sulfate solution is preferred, as sugar and salt solutions may distort the cysts. Diarrheic animals should be examined by direct smear for trophozoites; cyst forms will not be present.

There are no specific clinical signs in infected guinea pigs, but mucoid diarrhea has been reported in other infected rodents. *Giardia caviae* is not considered a public health problem.

Tritrichomonas caviae, like *Entamoeba caviae*, is mentioned in this chapter so that the technician can be aware that it is of little or no pathologic significance. Like *Tritrichomonas muris*, discussed in the mouse section, *T caviae* has 3 cranial flagella, and a free caudal flagellum. *Tritrichomonas caviae* (10-22 x 6-11 μ) is larger than *G caviae* and has an undulating membrane that extends the length of the body. The organisms are usually found in the cecum of guinea pigs. The technician should be aware that in cases of diarrhea produced by another cause, *T caviae* organisms proliferate secondarily, due to the fluid medium provided by the diarrhea. *Tritrichomonas caviae*, therefore, may be seen by direct fecal smear, particularly in animals with diarrhea.

Tritrichomonas caviae is transmitted between guinea pigs by ingestion of the trophozoites that have been passed in the feces of carrier animals. *Tritrichomonas caviae* is not seen in other species of animals and is not considered a public health hazard.

Sporozoa

Coccidia: Cryptosporidium wrairi of guinea pigs is similar to *C parvum* and *C muris*, previously discussed in the mouse section. However, *C wrairi* is considered a distinct species. Though oocysts of *C wrairi* have not been described, developing macrogametes are 4-7 μ in diameter and contain many refractile and polysaccharide granules.

Cryptosporidium wrairi is most commonly seen lining the tips of the intestinal villi in the ileum of young guinea pigs. Examination of fresh mucosal scrapings by phase-contrast microscopy may provide best results for detection and identification of *C wrairi.* Examination of paraffin-embedded materials is less satisfactory, especially when formalin is used as a fixative. The organisms appear extracellular, but actually are intracellular.

The only clinical sign of *C wrairi* infection is weight loss. Younger guinea pigs at 250-300 g are most likely to carry the parasite. Older animals seem to be resistant or have developed immunity to *C wrairi*. *Cryptosporidium wrairi* is not found in other species of animals and is not considered a public health problem.

Eimeria caviae is typical of the Eimeriorina, with an oval to slightly subspherical oocyst that is 13-26 x 12-23 μ. Oocyst walls are brownish and have no micropyle or polar granule. Oocysts, however, contain a residuum, as do sporocysts. *Eimeria caviae* is commonly found in the guinea pig's large intestine, particularly the ascending or proximal colon.

Eimeria caviae can be detected by fecal flotation. Repeated flotations should be done 4-5 days apart for 2-3 weeks. Diagnosis is made more consistently postmortem, where intestinal scrapings placed into saline may be examined microscopically for both intracellular stages and oocysts of *E caviae*.

Eimeria caviae is generally nonpathogenic, but young animals stressed by poor nutrition and husbandry may show clinical signs. Clinical signs are limited to diarrhea seen 11-13 days after exposure. The diarrhea ceases after a few days, if the animal is not reinfected. Diarrhea may continue if reinfection occurs.

As for the other species of *Eimeria*, *E caviae* is species specific, and so does not infect other species, including people.

PARASITES OF RABBITS
External Parasites

Fleas

Fleas are small, wingless insects with laterally flattened bodies. They are distinguished by large hind legs, which enable them to leap relatively great distances. Though specific hosts are preferred by different species of fleas, fleas are not necessarily host specific. In the absence of the preferred host, they readily attack another species for blood feeding. For this reason, flea infestation of rabbits will be discussed in general, rather than by particular species of fleas.

Fleas vary in size from 1 to 9 mm long and can usually be seen grossly by careful examination of the haircoat. The eggs are oval and white. They have no sticky coating and therefore are not often found on a host animal. As in other species, such as dogs and cats, flea droppings are a more common sign of flea infestation than the fleas themselves.

When flea infestation is suspected, a complete exam of the rabbit coat should be done, as different fleas prefer different parts of the body of the host. Some, such as *Cediopsylla simplex*, the common Eastern rabbit flea, are found around the face and neck, while others, such as *Odontopsyllus multispinosus*, the giant Eastern rabbit flea, are found over the tail head.

Fleas live most of their life off the host animal. Adults can easily leap distances of 7 feet to attack a host for a blood meal. Rabbits may be an alternate host when other indoor pets are treated for fleas. Fleas should be considered a public health hazard, as they act as vectors of several zoonotic diseases, including Rocky Mountain spotted fever and tularemia.

Flies

Larvae of some *Cuterebra* flies may encyst in the subcutaneous tissues of rabbits, as well as dogs, cats, mice, and occasionally people. After the eggs of *Cuterebra* hatch on the ground and become infective, larvae are ingested by the host rabbit. Depending on the particular species of *Cuterebra*, the larvae migrate to the area of preference in the subcutaneous tissue of the rabbit. As the larva matures, a breathing hole or fistula is formed to connect the encysted "bot" with the outside environment. The encysted *Cuterebra* bot may go unnoticed until the third-stage (final) larva is formed, at which time it may be seen through the fistula created in the skin and the encysted area may be easily palpated. When full grown in the host, *Cuterebra* bots may be up to 30 mm long and of a dark color (Fig 29). Usually there is an inflammatory reaction around the cyst that resolves within

10 days after the larva drops out of the host. However, secondary infection may develop and should be anticipated.

Cuterebra is transmitted by ingestion of infective larvae or possibly by penetration of the host skin by infective larvae. *Cuterebra* infection is rare in people, and the parasite cannot be transmitted directly to people through the encysted larva.

Lice

Hemodipsus ventricosis is uncommon but can be extremely debilitating to infested rabbits. *Hemodipsus ventricosis* is an Anopluran louse with narrow mouth parts specialized for sucking blood from the host. It has a small forebody and large rounded abdomen, with numerous long hairs. *Hemodipsus ventricosis* adults are 1.2-2.5 mm long and can be found antemortem by careful visual inspection of the haircoat, especially on the dorsal and lateral surfaces of the rabbit. Postmortem, hair may be pulled and placed in a Petri dish under a warm lamp and examined with a dissecting microscope or a hand-held magnifying glass. Adult lice are drawn by the warmth of the lamp to the tips of the hair. The nits of *H ventricosis* are oval and 0.5-0.7 mm long. They may be found attached to the base of hair shafts by pulling the fur and examining microscopically.

Clinical signs of *H ventricosis* infestation include alopecia and ruffled fur. Rabbit lice are avid bloodsuckers, so anemia may occur in severe infestations.

Hemodipsus ventricosis is transmitted from rabbit to rabbit by prolonged direct contact. This mostly occurs between a doe

Figure 29. *Cuterebra* bot, the larva of a *Cuterebra* fly.

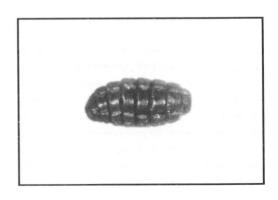

and her litter. Though *H ventricosis* is not considered zoonotic, it is a vector of *Franciscella tularensis*, the cause of tularemia.

Burrowing Mites

Rabbits can be infested by notoedric and sarcoptic mange mites. Both cause similar lesions usually on the head, neck and legs. Lesions may also appear on the pinnae, making it necessary to distinguish *Notoedres cati* (Fig 15) and *Sarcoptes scabiei* (Fig 16) from the rabbit ear mite, *Psoroptes cuniculi* (Fig 30).

In general, notoedric mites are smaller than sarcoptic mites, and *P cuniculi* is larger than both. Except for size, the major distinguishing characteristic of *N cati* and *S scabiei* is location of the mite's anus. The anus is dorsal in notoedric mites and terminal in sarcoptic mites. In notoedric and sarcoptic mites, suckers are found at the end of unjointed stalks on the first 2 pairs of legs in adult females, and on the first, second and fourth pairs of legs in adult males. Psoroptic mites are distinguished by suckers at the end of jointed stalks on the first, second and fourth pairs of legs in females, and the first, second and third pairs of legs in males.

Diagnosis of *N cati* or *S scabiei* infestation is by identification of adult parasites or eggs from deep skin scrapings. Deep skin

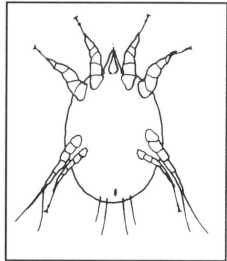

Figure 30. Line drawing of a *Psoroptes cuniculi* female, the rabbit ear mite.

scrapings from the edges of lesions are necessary to detect the burrowing mites. Lesions normally begin near the nose or lips and spread over the face, and may eventually involve the external or lateral pinna, the extremities, and genital region. Both *N cati* and *S scabiei* cause intense pruritus that may result in self-mutilation. A crust or scale may develop over infested areas, and the skin may become thick and wrinkled. Secondary bacterial infection is not uncommon.

Transmission of notoedric and sarcoptic mange mites is by direct contact.

Ear Mites

Psoroptes cuniculi, the rabbit ear mite, is probably the most common ectoparasite of rabbits. These nonburrowing mites pierce the epidermis of the ear to feed on tissue fluids. A scab then forms and the mites live under the scab.

Psoroptes cuniculi must be distinguished from burrowing mites because both kinds of burrowing mites and *Psoroptes* may be found on the ears of rabbits. Psoroptic mites are distinguished from notoedric and sarcoptic mites by the jointed stalks, or pedicles, on their legs, from which the suckers arise (Fig 30). Burrowing mites have unjointed pedicles. *Psoroptes cuniculi* mites of both sexes are relatively large. Females are 409-749 x 351-499 μ, and males are 431-547 x 322-462 μ. The mites can be seen with the unaided eye or with a hand-held magnifying glass.

Psoroptes cuniculi is found in the ears of rabbits with light brown, crusty material in the auditory canal and on the inner surfaces of the pinnae. The mites can be recovered on a cotton-tipped applicator that has been dipped in mineral oil and then examined microscopically for accurate identification.

Clinical signs associated with *P cuniculi* infestation include head shaking, ear scratching, and formation of a brownish crust in the ear canal. In advanced cases, this crusty material may actually appear like a plug in the ear canal, as well as lining the pinnae. Though commonly associated with otitis media produced by secondary infection with *Pasteurella multocida*, the ear mites themselves are not responsible for this condition. Transmission of *P cuniculi* is by direct contact. There is no cross species contamination or zoonotic potential.

Fur Mites

Cheyletiella parasitivorax (Fig 31) and *Listrophorus gibbus* are small, oval, nonburrowing fur mites of rabbits. Cheyletid mites are more common, especially in domestic rabbits. These small, oval mites are characterized by the large, curved hooks or palpi on either side of the mouth. Adult females are 350-500 μ long. Adult males are about 285 μ long. *Listrophorus gibbus* females are about 435 μ and males 340 μ long. Both have a dorsal hood-like projection that covers the mouthparts. Males are further characterized by the clasping organs at their caudal end.

Both types of rabbit fur mites may be detected by pulling fur with a forceps or with cellophane tape, and then examining under a dissecting microscope. Combing or brushing the fur may also be used to obtain mites for identification. *Cheyletiella parasitivorax* mites are most likely located dorsally, between or near the shoulders, and *L gibbus* on the back and abdomen. Body

Figure 31. *Cheyletiella parasitivorax,* the common fur mite of rabbits.

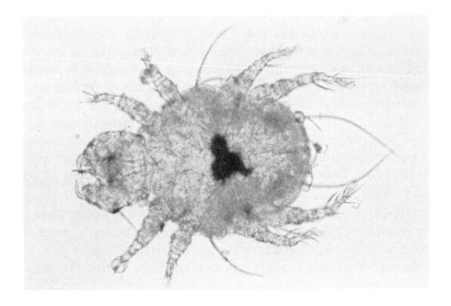

areas to examine for *C parasitivorax* in particular may have partial alopecia, with underlying reddened skin and a fine whitish crusty material that resembles dandruff. Fur can be pulled in clumps from these areas. Though infested skin is painful to the touch, affected rabbits usually show no signs of pruritus from *C parasitivorax* infestation. Light infestations often go unnoticed. *Listrophorus gibbus* appears to produce no clinical signs, even in heavy infestations.

Both rabbit fur mites are transmitted by direct contact. *Listrophorus gibbus* is more commonly associated with wild rabbits than with domestic rabbits, so owners should be aware that control of this parasite depends on controlling the rabbit's environment. *Listrophorus gibbus* is not a known vector of disease, including zoonoses. *Cheyletiella parasitivorax* can transmit myxomatosis among rabbits and has produced dermatitis in dogs, cats and people. Technicians should use caution when handling infested rabbits.

Ticks

Though numerous kinds of ticks may infest rabbits, most have a limited geographic distribution and are generally recognized by technicians working in each geographic location. This discussion will center on the continental rabbit tick, *Hemaphysalis leporis*, which has the widest geographic distribution of rabbit ticks in the Western Hemisphere. *Hemaphysalis leporis* is a 3-host tick, meaning that each stage (larva, nymph, adult) requires a separate host for a blood meal. Though rabbits may serve as the host for each stage, they seem to be the definitive host for only the adult stage. Larval and nymphal stages also feed on birds, occasionally on dogs and cats, and rarely on people. Feeding on birds is thought to account for much of the wide geographic distribution of *H leporis*, as the birds are often migratory.

Hemaphysalis leporis is a small, eyeless tick, and is distinguished in all stages of the life cycle by the laterally pointed angles formed at the base of the mouthparts. These angles, or capituli, cause the mouthparts to resemble a triangular head. Males are 2.2 mm long and females are 2.6-10.0 mm long, depending on whether they are engorged with blood. The ticks may be found in the ear canal and on the pinnae, but are more frequently seen on the head and neck.

Ticks are voracious blood feeders that normally drop off the host after a blood meal, so few are found on the host at one time. In extreme cases, large numbers of ticks may cause emaciation and death. As with many tick infestations, the primary concern with rabbit tick infestation is transmission of disease, such as Rocky Mountain spotted fever, Q fever and tularemia. In general, ticks are more common on wild than domestic rabbits, so owners should be warned of the disease potential both to rabbits and people if domestic rabbits are not kept safely away from all types of wild rabbits and birds.

Internal Parasites

Tapeworms

Domestic rabbits and wild cottontail rabbits, wild hares and wild rodents may act as intermediate hosts in the life cycle of the carnivore tapeworm, *Taenia pisiformis*. The larval form found in the peritoneal cavity of rabbits is referred to as *Cysticercus pisiformis*. The adult worm from carnivores (usually dogs) is passed in the feces as gravid (egg-bearing) proglottids and/or eggs. Gravid proglottids are cream colored, and longer than wide (9.5 x 4.5 mm). Eggs from the proglottids are dark brown and nearly spherical (32 x 37 μ). Rabbits acquire infections by ingesting feed, bedding or other materials contaminated by proglottids or eggs. Taenid eggs then hatch in the small intestine of the rabbit and migrate through the liver for about one month. When the larvae reach the surface of the liver, they are 1-2 cm in diameter and resemble a clear, whitish cyst. The larva may then leave the liver and attach to viscera or mesenteric surfaces in the peritoneal cavity. Carnivores are reinfected by ingesting abdominal viscera from infected rabbits.

Infection with *C pisiformis* is not usually diagnosed until liver lesions or the larval forms in the abdominal cavity are seen at necropsy of the rabbit. Heavy infections may be suspected in live rabbits presented with a pot-bellied appearance, weight loss and lethargy. Clients should be advised to prevent fecal contamination of rabbit feed and bedding by carnivores, and to deworm dogs and cats in the household.

The life cycle of *Multiceps serialis* or the larval stage, *Coernus serialis*, is analogous to that of *T pisiformis*, except in its location in the intermediate host. *Multiceps serialis* larvae develop in subcutaneous tissues and skeletal muscles of rabbits, as opposed to the liver and abdominal cavity in the case of *T pisiformis*. Antemortem detection may be by observation and palpation of the cyst-like larval enlargements. Neither of these tapeworms has zoonotic potential, but they must be controlled by careful storage of feed and bedding of rabbits and regular deworming of dogs and cats, especially those with free outdoor access.

Nematodes

Oxyurids (Pinworms): Passalurus ambiguus is a nonpathogenic pinworm found in the cecum and colon of domestic and cottontail rabbits and hares. It is typically oxyurid in appearance, having an obvious round esophageal bulb. Adult females are about 10 mm long (Fig 32) and males are 4-5 mm long (Fig 33). Females have a long, finely pointed tail. Ova are oval and slightly flattened on one side, measuring about 43 x 103 μ (Fig 34). Ova deposited in the feces are morulated like hookworm ova of dogs.

Antemortem, *P ambiguus* infection can be detected by observing ova in fecal flotation preparations. Postmortem, the white hair-like adult worms can be found in the cecum and proximal colon. Rabbits can tolerate heavy infections with no apparent clinical signs. It is thought that pinworms feed on bacteria in the intestinal contents without disturbing the mucosal lining of the cecum.

Ova passed in the feces are immediately infective, so control of this parasite is difficult. Transmission is by ingestion of infective ova. Clients should be advised to use feeders elevated off of the floor of the rabbit hutch and to prevent wild hare and cottontail access to pet rabbits and their feed and bedding. *Passalurus ambiguus* is species specific and has no zoonotic potential.

Figure 32. Adult female *Passalurus ambiguus*. Note the long slender tail.

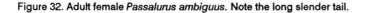

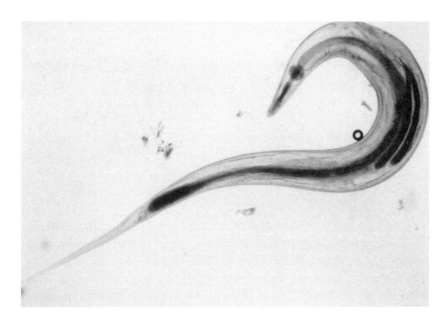

Figure 32. Adult female *Passalurus ambiguus*. Note the long slender tail.

Trichostrongyles: Though these nematodes are generally common in wild and uncommon in domestic rabbits, technicians should be aware of the possibility of infection with one or more rabbit trichostrongyles. *Obeliscoides cuniculi* adults are found in the stomach of rabbits, while adults of *Trichostrongylus*

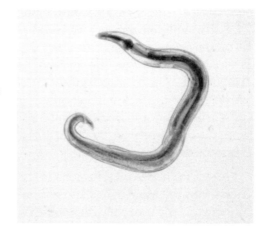

Figure 33. Adult male *Passalurus ambiguus*.

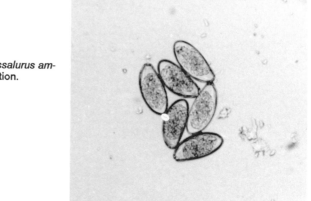

Figure 34. Ova of *Passalurus ambiguus* in a fecal flotation.

calcaratus are found in the small intestine. The males of these species are distinguished by the cuticular bursa copulatrix, which is supported by rays at the caudal end of the body. *Obeliscoides cuniculi* females are 16 mm long x 0.5 mm wide, and males are 12 x 0.2 mm. Male and female adults may be found in the stomach postmortem. Ova are 80 x 45 μ, thin-shelled and oval, and can be seen in fecal flotation preparations. This nematode can cause hemorrhagic gastritis. Transmission is by ingestion of the larval form developed after eggs are passed in the feces.

Adults of *T calcaratus* are found in the small intestine and generally are smaller than those of *O cuniculi*. Females of *T calcaratus* are 6.4 mm x 100 μ and males are 5.7 mm x 115 μ. The thin-shelled ova are 65 x 33 μ and may be seen in fecal flotation preparations. Rabbits infected with *T calcaratus* may develop anemia. The life cycle of the nematode is direct, and transmission is by ingestion of infective larvae. As with other parasites that infect wild rabbits, prevention and control depend on storing feed and bedding safely from wild animal access.

Sporozoa

Intestinal Coccidia: Numerous species of *Eimeria* coccidia can infect rabbits. Most affect the gut, and one, *E steidae*, affects the bile ducts. The more pathogenic *Eimeria* spp that affect the gut will be discussed here; *E steidae* will be considered separately. The intestinal coccidia of rabbits include *E irresidua, E magna, E media* and *E perforans*. All *Eimeria* spp affect the small intestine; *E media* may also affect the large intestine.

The oocysts of *E irresidua* are 38 x 26 μ and ovoid. The wall of the oocyst is smooth and light yellow. There is a wide micropyle, with no polar granules or residuum. Sporocysts within the oocyst are also ovoid, with both a Steida body and residuum. Antemortem diagnosis depends on recognition of the mature oocyst, along with clinical signs, which may include severe hemorrhagic diarrhea, excessive thirst and dehydration. Postmortem indications include inflammation of the intestines and sloughing of the gut lining.

The mature oocyst of *E magna* is 35 x 24 μ and ovoid, with a distinctive dark yellow-brown wall (Fig 35). A wide micropyle appears built up around the rim, with no micropyle cap. Oocysts and sporocysts (Fig 36) contain a residuum. The sporocysts are ovoid and have a Steida body. *Eimeria magna*, like *E irresidua*, is highly pathogenic. Clinical signs include weight loss, anorexia and mucoid diarrhea. Necropsy signs include inflammation and sloughing of the gut lining.

Eimeria media oocysts are ovoid and 31 x 18 μ, with a smooth wall and light pink color. There is a micropyle and a residuum. Sporocysts within the mature oocyst are ovoid, with a Steida body and a residuum. *Eimeria media* is moderately pathogenic

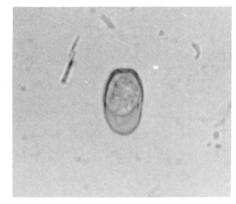

Figure 35. Unsporulated oocyst of the rabbit intestinal coccidian, *Eimeria magna.*

and may cause enteritis and diarrhea. At necropsy, the intestinal wall may be edematous and contain gray foci of necrosis.

Eimeria perforans is the least pathogenic rabbit coccidian to be discussed. Oocysts are ovoid and 21 x 15 μ with a smooth wall, no micropyle and a small residuum. Oocysts appear distinctly smaller than those of other *Eimeria* spp in mixed infections. Sporocysts within the mature oocyst are ovoid, with a Steida body and residuum. Mild diarrhea may be seen. Postmortem changes may include an edematous, whitish duodenum, and multiple white spots and streaks in the jejunum and ileum.

Transmission of coccidia is by ingestion of sporulated oocysts. After ingestion, the prepatent periods range from 5 days for *E perforans* to 8 days for *E irresidua*. Antemortem detection for all *Eimeria* spp is by direct fecal smear and fecal flotation preparation examination for oocysts. It may be necessary to retain coccidia-positive feces for 3-5 days to allow sporulation of oocysts, making positive species identification possible. Coccidia-positive fecal material may be placed in 2% potassium dichromate solution, which fixes the fecal material and enhances sporulation of oocysts.

Liver Coccidia: Eimeria steidae is a highly pathogenic coccidian that affects the bile ducts of rabbits. It causes variable mortality, which is highest in young rabbits. Oocysts of *E steidae* are 35 x 20 μ and ovoid, with a flattened pole at the micropyle

Figure 36. *Eimeria magna* oocyst after sporulation. The arrow indicates the micropyle. The round darkened body in the center is the residuum. The 4 oval lighter bodies are sporocysts.

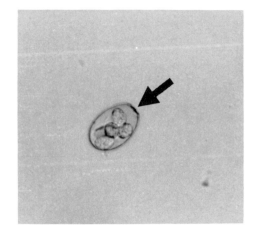

end. The wall is smooth and yellow. There is no polar granule or residuum. Sporocysts are ovoid, with a Steida body and a residuum.

Light infections usually produce no clinical signs. Heavier infections may cause blockage of the bile ducts and impaired liver function, resulting in icterus and a distended abdomen due to liver enlargement. Diarrhea or constipation and anorexia may be noted. At necropsy, white, dilated nodules are likely to be seen in the liver. Hyperplastic bile ducts contain a yellow-green creamy material, in which oocysts may be seen in impression smears when examined microscopically. Transmission of *E steidae* is by ingestion of sporulated oocysts passed in the feces. The prepatent period is 15-18 days. As in all *Eimeria* species, there is no cross species contamination or public health importance.

References

Flynn: *Parasites of Laboratory Animals*. 1st ed. Iowa State University Press, Ames, 1973.

Harkness and Wagner: *The Biology and Medicine of Rabbits and Rodents*. 3rd ed. Lea & Febiger, Philadelphia, 1989.

Hsu, in Baker *et al: The Laboratory Rat. Vol I, Biology and Diseases*. Academic Press, Orlando, 1979.

Hsu, in Foster: *The Mouse in Biomedical Research*. Vol II. Academic Press, New York, 1982.

Kraus, in Weisbroth *et al: The Biology of the Laboratory Rabbit*. Academic Press, Orlando, 1974.

Pakes, in Weisbroth *et al: The Biology of the Laboratory Rabbit*. Academic Press, Orlando, 1974.

Ronald and Wagner, in Wagner and Manning: *The Biology of the Laboratory Guinea Pig*. Academic Press, Orlando, 1976.

Sloss and Kemp: *Veterinary Clinical Parasitology*. 5th ed. Iowa State University Press, Ames, 1978.

Vetterling, in Wagner and Manning: *The Biology of the Laboratory Guinea Pig*. Academic Press, Orlando, 1976.

Wagner, in Van Hoosier and McPherson: *The Laboratory Hamster*. Academic Press, Orlando, 1987.

Westcott, in Wagner and Manning: *The Biology of the Laboratory Guinea Pig*. Academic Press, New York, 1976.

Westcott, in Weisbroth *et al: The Biology of the Laboratory Rabbit*. Academic Press, Orlando, 1974.

10

Parasites of Pet and Aviary Birds

A. M. Fudge

Pet and aviary birds are the most common type of avian patient treated by the veterinarian. Other types of avian patients include backyard poultry, waterfowl and wild birds.

Parasites are not common in many species of pet birds. For example, endoparasites and ectoparasites in the popular Amazon Parrots are extremely rare, indicating that fecal flotations for this group of birds are not of great value. Some imported birds harbor parasitic infections that can be intensified in a captive breeding facility. Australian Grass Parakeets (Bourke's, Rosellas) frequently are infected with roundworms when kept in aviary. Giardiasis is very common in Cockatiels and Budgerigars. Ectoparasites of pet birds are also rare, with a few exceptions.

Backyard poultry and waterfowl are commonly infected with endoparasites and should be checked regularly. It is rare *not* to find parasites in a group of these birds.

Wild birds are often hosts for a wide variety of parasites. Parasitism in healthy wild birds is normal. When a wild bird becomes a captive, however, parasite loads can increase and become important clinically.

Techniques to Identify Avian Parasites

External Parasites

With few exceptions, external parasites are rare in pet birds. Skin scrapings for mites are useful when examining certain avian species. Care must be taken when making a scraping, as avian skin tears easily and usually has little subcutaneous padding.

External feather parasites can be grasped with forceps or killed with an appropriate pesticide to allow closer examination.

External parasites may be examined under the low-power objective of the microscope. Place the parasite on the slide, then add mineral oil or immersion oil. Place a coverslip over this preparation. You may also use mounting cement in place of mineral oil.

Internal Parasites

Direct fecal smears should always be performed when assessing a bird for parasites. Flotation using sodium nitrate solutions can be useful when looking for ova. Flagellates are common in some avian species, but are not seen in a flotation. In our laboratory, the trichrome stain is employed to improve the probability of finding flagellates, such as *Giardia*, in susceptible species (Table 1). The very fresh fecal sample is placed in polyvinyl alcohol (PVA) for preservation. Then the sample is smeared on the slide, incubated and stained.

Blood Parasites

Blood parasites are usually identified in blood smears prepared for hematologic assessment. I prefer a quick Wright's-type stain for avian hematology. Extracellular parasites (microfilariae, *Trypanosoma*) tend to be found at the periphery of blood smears. Examination of the buffy coat smears increases the possibility of finding these parasites. Alternatively, you can examine the intact hematocrit tube under the low-power objective of the microscope. Focus on the plasma/cell interface and look for motile forms of these parasites.

Table 1. Fecal trichrome staining procedure for flagellate endoparasites.

Solutions

Polyvinyl alcohol fixative (PVA): Purchase stock solution.

Iodine alcohol: Stock solution is prepared by dissolving iodine crystals in 70% ethanol. To obtain solution suitable for staining, dilute the stock solution with 70% ethanol until a port wine color is obtained.

Trichrome stain: Purchase stock solution; making from scratch is costly.

Acid Alcohol: Glacial acetic acid 0.45 ml, 90% ethanol 99.55 ml.

Carbol xylene: Because of restriction on shipping, using and storing phenol, carbol xylene solution should be purchased.

Staining Procedure

Remove PVA-fixed feces and smear 2-3 drops onto a slide with an applicator. Incubate the slides overnight at 37 C. It is best to use covered Coplin jars to immerse the slides in staining solutions:

1. Iodine alcohol: 10-20 minutes
2. Ethanol 70%: 3-5 minutes (first immersion)
3. Ethanol 70%: 3-5 minutes (second immersion)
4. Trichrome: 6-8 minutes
5. Acid alcohol: 10-20 seconds
6. Ethanol 95%: Rinse
7. Ethanol 95%: 5 minutes
8. Carbol xylene: 5-10 minutes
9. Xylene: 10 minutes
10. Mount with coverslip (optional because it is difficult to mount thick smears)

External Parasites

Mites

Mites are commonly found on backyard poultry. The northern fowl mite, *Ornithonyssus* spp (Fig 1), remains on the host. *Dermanyssus* spp, the red mite of poultry, feeds on the birds at night, spending most of its time off of the bird. Feather mites of caged birds are apparently rare in North America. I have seen only 2 cases in 12 years of pet bird practice: a Cockatiel caged with an apparently ineffective and unnecessary "mite protector," and a Canary recently imported from the Netherlands. Apparently these mites are a clinical problem in Western European Canaries. You should not spend a lot of time looking for these parasites in pet birds, but you will have the opportunity

Figure 1. Northern fowl mite removed from a chicken.

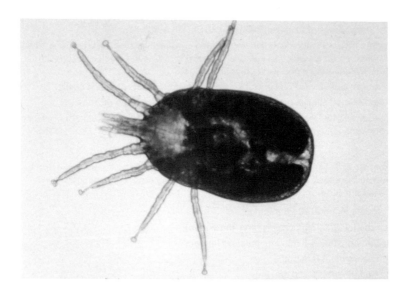

to see them when treating backyard poultry, waterfowl and selected wild birds.

Feather quill mites (*Syringophilus* spp) are occasionally found within the feather follicle of Cockatoos. A squash preparation of a feather quill may demonstrate these mites. A surgical skin and follicle biopsy most frequently diagnose these parasites and is most useful for evaluating other more common causes of feather problems. In pet bird species other than Cockatoos, feather quill mites are apparently rare.

Skin mites occur in selected pet bird species. The best known is *Knemidocoptes* spp (Fig 2), the causative agent of scaly leg/scaly face in Budgerigars and tasselfoot in Canaries. *Knemidocoptes* is also found in the Kakariki, an Australian Parrot and occasionally other Parrots with immunodeficiencies. Characteristic signs include skin thickening characterized by a white honeycomb type layer. In Canaries, proliferation and thickening of the toes and feet can be caused by the same type of parasite. *Knemidocoptes* is also found in poultry and wild birds.

Figure 2. *Knemidocoptes*, the cause of scaly face/scaly leg in Budgerigars and tasselfoot in Canaries.

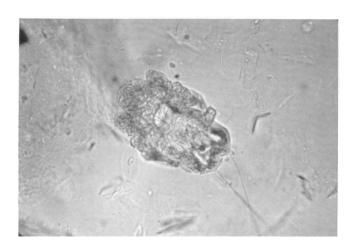

Mange mites are seen rather uniquely in one popular species of pet bird, the Gray-Cheeked Parakeet (*Brotogeris pyrrhopteruss*). It causes pruritus and flaking, and can be demonstrated in skin scrapings of affected areas (Fig 3).

Figure 3. Mange mite (*Acuaria?*) in a skin scraping taken from a Gray-Cheeked Parakeet.

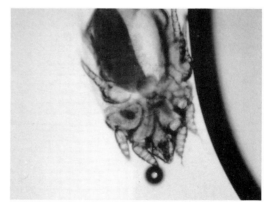

Lice

Biting lice are rarely found in pet birds and seem to be most common in Cockatiels from infested aviaries (Figs 4-6). While infestation can become heavy, clinical problems, such as pruri-

Figure 4. A biting feather louse found on a Parrot. This rare finding was from a group of recently imported Parrots dying of a viral disease and submitted for necropsy.

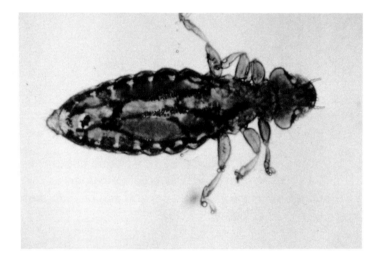

Figure 5. A biting feather louse removed from a Cockatiel. Lice infrequently infest Cockatiel aviaries. They are found on the wings and tail feathers of infested birds.

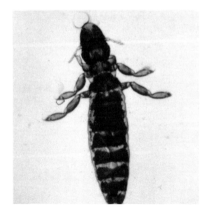

Figure 6. A biting feather louse removed from a Magpie.

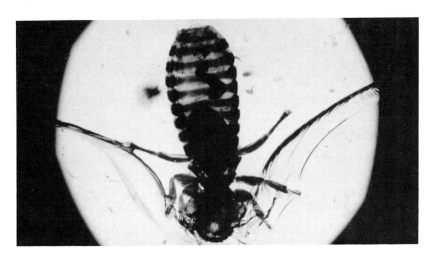

tus, are uncommon. Lice are commonly found in a large number of backyard poultry/waterfowl and wild birds.

Mosquitos, Flies, Ticks, Fleas

Other parasites can be a local problem in selected birds. Mosquitos can transmit *Plasmodium* to Canaries kept in out-

Figure 7. A sticktight flea removed from a chicken.

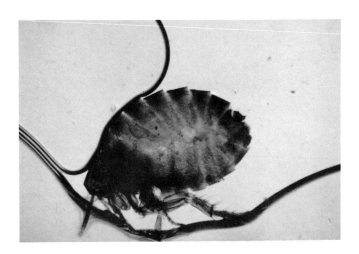

door aviaries. Hippoboscid flies are found on wild birds and can transmit blood parasites. Ticks have been reported in some aviary collections but are rare in pet birds. The sticktight flea of poultry (Fig 7) firmly attaches itself around the head and eyes of the bird and can infest domestic mammals.

Respiratory Tract Parasites

Air Sac Mites

Air sac mites (*Sternastoma tracheacolum*) are common in Canaries and selected species of Finches, particularly the Lady Gouldian Finch. These parasites reside in the trachea and airways, where their activity can lead to pneumonia. Contrary to general belief, mite eggs are not often found in the stool. Diagnosis usually requires visualization in the trachea by transillumination, finding the mites at necropsy, or response to therapy. Air sac mites have been visualized in Parrots during laparoscopic sex determination procedures and have not been usually associated with clinical disease in such cases.

Gapeworms

The gapeworm (*Syngamus trachea)* and related species live in the trachea and major airways of poultry, waterfowl and selected wild birds. The ova can be seen in fecal samples (Fig 8).

Figure 8. A gapeworm (*Syngamus trachea*) ovum in a fecal smear from a Hawaiian Snow Goose.

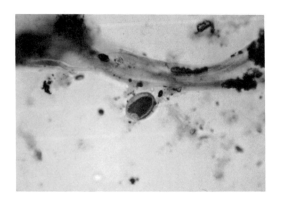

Atoxoplasma

Atoxoplasma serini is a protozoan parasite of Canaries and Finches (Fig 9). *Atoxoplasma* can affect a number of organs, causing respiratory signs. The parasite is best visualized on organ impression smears of the lung, liver and spleen.

Alimentary Tract Parasites

Helminths

Roundworms occur infrequently in caged birds. *Ascardia* is occasionally seen in Lovebirds, Cockatiels and Macaws (Fig 10). It is very common in Grass Parakeets and can be demonstrated

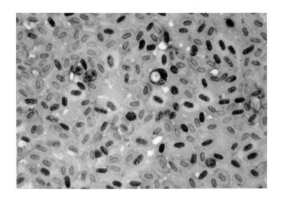

Figure 9. *Atoxoplasma serini* in a mononuclear cell on a lung impression smear from a Canary. (Wright's stain)

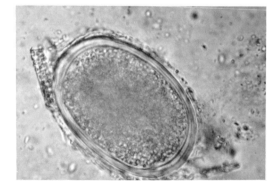

Figure 10. A roundworm (*Ascaridia*) ovum in a fecal smear from a Cockatiel.

in direct smears and fecal flotations. Roundworms are common in backyard poultry and waterfowl (Fig 11). In Turkeys and Peafowl, *Heterakis gallinarum* serves as the intermediate host for the liver protozoan, *Histomonas meleagridis*.

Spirurids (gizzard worms) can infect a variety of avian species but are generally uncommon in pet birds. *Spiroptera incesta* can infect Australian Parakeets. *Dispharynx nasuta* can infect Finches.

Spirurid infections can be difficult to detect by fecal examination in Finches. When this parasite is suspected, histologic examination of the ventriculus is recommended. Spirurid eggs are characterized by their thick wall and embryonated contents.

Tetrameres is most commonly found in Pigeons, in the wall of the proventriculus.

Capillaria spp (threadworms) occur in the crop and upper alimentary tract. They are common in Pheasants, Peafowl and poultry. *Capillaria* infections have been reported in imported psittacine birds. The small adult worm can often be found in the wall of the esophagus or crop. A direct smear of a sample from this area or a fecal flotation shows the characteristic thick-walled oval bipolar ova (Fig 12), which are similar to those of whipworms in carnivores.

Tapeworms are common in imported Cockatoos and African Parrots. Because whole proglottids are shed, fecal flotations rarely demonstrate tapeworm ova. Eosinophilia seems to be

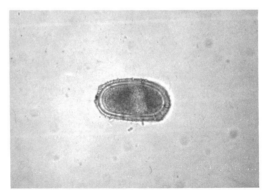

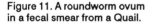
Figure 11. A roundworm ovum in a fecal smear from a Quail.

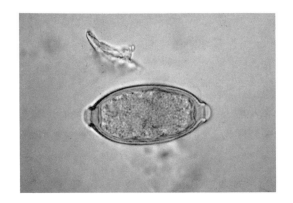

Figure 12. *Capillaria* ovum in a direct fecal smear from a Macaw.

associated with tapeworm infections in Parrots. In Australian Finches, tapeworm infections can become quite severe and may cause death.

Protozoa

Giardia is the most common protozoan seen in pet bird practice. This flagellated parasite is most commonly found in Cockatiels, Budgerigars and Lovebirds. The feces of affected birds often become voluminous and chunky, with a pea-soup consistency. Fresh saline direct mounts can demonstrate the trophozoites, with characteristic "falling leaf" motility. Allergic skin conditions may be associated with giardiasis in Cockatiels. It may be difficult to demonstrate *Giardia* in some of these cases.

The fecal trichrome stain can enhance visualization of the parasite (Fig 13). Other stains used to enhance visualization include Lugol's iodine, Gram's iodine and Wright's stain. In my experience, other stains may incidentally demonstrate trophozoites, such as acid-fast stain or Gram's stain (Fig 14).

Histomonas meleagridis infects Turkeys and Peafowl, causing severe and fatal liver disease (blackhead). Diagnosis is usually by histologic examination of the liver. Suspicion of infection is increased by finding the ova of the worm *Heterakis gallinarum* in the feces.

Trichomonas gallinae is frequently found in crop washes and crop swabs of Pigeons, Doves and poultry. Occasionally this

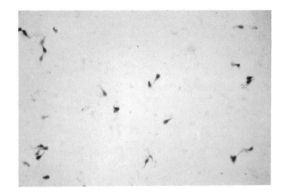

Figure 13. *Giardia* trophozoites. (trichrome stain)

parasite is associated with Finch mortality. In North America, trichomoniasis appears to be rare in psittacine birds but has been reported in Budgerigars. The parasite is best demonstrated by a direct saline smear of crop contents and is characterized by 4 cranial flagella. An air-dried smear can be stained with Wright's stain. The parasite assumes an oval shape, staining blue with a red axostyle (Fig 15).

Coccidial infections are rare in pet birds, though *Isospora* and *Eimeria* have been reported. Coccidia are commonly found in Pigeons and poultry. A common error made by inexperienced technicians is to mistake normal urate crystals for coccidia (Fig 16). A related sporozoan, *Atoxoplasma serini*, which can infect Canaries and Finches, has lung-liver, blood and intestinal forms (Fig 9). The intestinal form is small and hard to find. *Cryptosporidium* has been found in Cockatiels. This tiny sporozoan

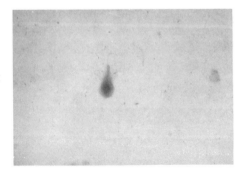

Figure 14. A *Giardia* trophozoite, showing flagellar detail, in a Gram-stained fecal smear. This was an incidental finding, as Gram stain is not the stain of choice for flagellates.

Figure 15. *Trichomonas gallinae* in a crop wash from a Dove.

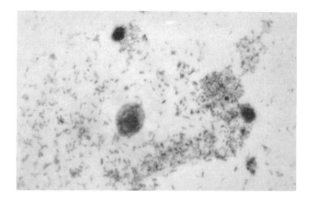

parasite is also difficult to visualize in fecal samples and is usually diagnosed by histologic examination of the intestine.

Blood Parasites

Blood parasites are common in pet birds. In most cases they cause little clinical disease. Finding and reporting these parasites demonstrate the skill of the technician performing an avian hematologic study.

Figure 16. Urate crystals in an avian urine sample. These are frequently mistaken for fecal parasites, such as coccidia, by inexperienced technicians.

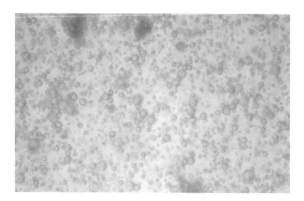

Hemoproteus is commonly found in the erythrocytes of the white species of Cockatoos, Green-Winged Macaws, and some species of Conures. This blood parasite is rarely associated with clinical disease, such as anemia. *Hemoproteus* is characterized by a bluish sausage shape in the cytoplasm, sometimes overlaid with blue dots (Fig 17). It infects a variety of wild waterfowl and can cause death in these birds.

Plasmodium (malaria) causes mortality in Canaries in some parts of the country. This may be due to transmission of a local passerine strain via mosquitos to susceptible Canaries. The organism may not be present in the peripheral blood. A "signet ring" form, in which the cytoplasm displaces the erythrocyte nucleus, is the most common form seen (Fig 18). Diagnosis of *Plasmodium* infections is also by organ impression smears and histopathologic examination of the liver and spleen.

Leucocytozoon infects the leukocytes of birds of prey (Owls, Hawks, Falcons), greatly distorting the shape and appearance of the leukocyte. A variety of forms can be present and can be associated with occasional leukocytosis and disease. The most common morphology is the fusiform or spindle shape (Fig 19).

Figure 17. *Hemoproteus* is normally seen as a sausage-shaped body in the cytoplasm of the avian erythrocyte.

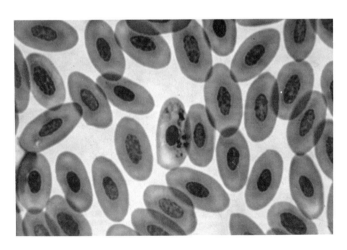

Figure 18. *Plasmodium* displacing the nucleus of erythrocytes in the blood of a Canary.

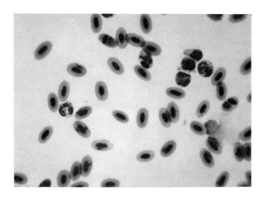

Figure 19. *Leucocytozoon* in the blood of a Red-Tailed Hawk.

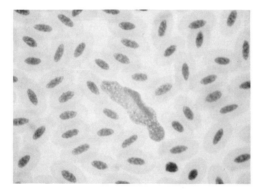

Aegyptianella is occasionally found in pet birds. I have seen the parasite in African Gray Parrots, in which it caused little clinical problem. The parasite infects the erythrocyte, appearing as a marginated dot on the cells.

Trypanosoma is occasionally found in Cockatoos and rarely causes clinical disease. The organism does not infect blood cells in the peripheral blood and has a very distinctive appearance (Fig 20).

Microfilariae are commonly found in Cockatoos and occasionally passerine birds. The adult filarid worm lives in the subcutaneous tissues or the serosal linings of the host, usually causing

Figure 20. *Trypanosoma* in the blood of a Cockatoo.

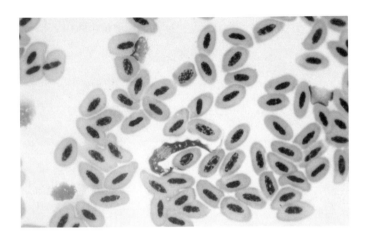

Figure 21. A microfilaria in the blood of a Cockatoo.

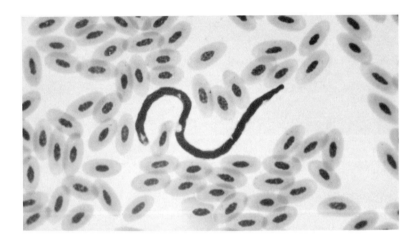

little disease. Occasionally the adult worm causes lung, heart, or skin disease. Microfilaremia (microfilariae in the blood) (Fig 21) is not usually associated with disease. No effective treatment is available to kill the adult worms.

Filarid worms occasionally infect the feet or toes of Parrots, causing inflammation and swelling. They are removed surgically (Fig 22). Microfilaremia is not a consistent finding.

Figure 22. A filarid worm surgically removed from the swollen toe of a Green-Winged Macaw.

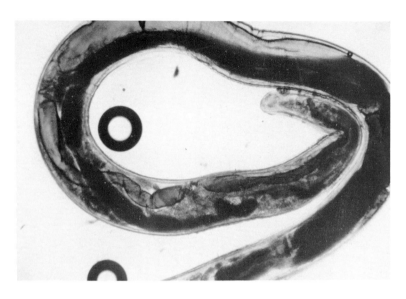

Recommended Reading

Barnes, in Harrison and Harrison: *Clinical Avian Medicine and Surgery.* Saunders, Philadelphia, 1986.

Campbell: *Avian Hematology and Cytology.* Iowa State University Press, Ames, 1988.

Flammer: Clinical aspects of atoxoplasmosis in Canaries. *Proc Ann Mtg Assn Avian Vet,* 1987. pp 33-36.

Fudge: Avian hematology: identification and interpretation. *Proc Ann Mtg Assn Avian Vet,* 1989. pp 284-292.

Fudge and McEntee: Avian giardiasis: syndromes, diagnosis and therapy. *Proc Ann Mtg Assn Avian Vet,* 1986. pp 155-164.

Keymer, in Petrak: *Diseases of Cage and Aviary Birds.* Lea & Febiger, Philadelphia, 1982.

McCluggage: Parasitology of caged birds. *Proc Ann Mtg Assn Avian Vet,* 1989. pp 97-100.

Orme: Common hematozoa in caged birds. *Proc Ann Conf Assn Avian Tech,* 1988. pp 1-16.

Glossary

Acariasis: Disease caused by a mite or tick.

Anorexia: Loss of appetite.

Arachnid: A member of the class Arachnida, which includes spiders, ticks and mites.

Arthropod: A member of the phylum Arthropoda, the largest animal phylum, which includes insects, arachnids and crustaceans.

Artifact: Anything artificially produced.

Ascariasis: Infection by roundworms.

Cestode: A tapeworm.

Coenurus: A cyst form of certain tapeworm species found in the intermediate host.

Cuticle: A layer of solid or semisolid substance that covers the free surface of a layer of epithelial cells.

Cysticercus: The encysted larval form of a tapeworm consisting of a rounded cyst or bladder into which the scolex is invaginated.

Dead-end host: A host that a parasite can infect, but in which no further parasite development, especially reproduction, occurs.

Decorticated: The state of a parasite egg with the outer shell removed.

Definitive host: The final host in which the parasite reaches sexual maturity.

Direct life cycle: A parasite life cycle requiring no intermediate host(s) for completion.

Ectoparasite: Parasite living on the body surface of its host.

Egg: Female reproductive cell.

Embryonated: Containing a developed nucleus. In parasitology, usually a larval form.

Enzootic: Disease that exists in an area, but only occurs sporadically.

Endoparasite: Parasite living within the body of the host.

Filariform: Cylindric esophageal structure without a bulb, found in certain larval stages and some adult parasites, especially *Strongyloides.*

Final host: Definitive host.

Flagellum: Hairlike, motile process on the extremity of a protozoan.

Indirect life cycle: Parasite life cycle requiring one or more intermediate hosts for completion.

Infective larva: Life cycle stage capable of causing a parasitic infection.

Infestation: The harboring of animal parasites, especially macroscopic forms, such as ectoparasites.

Intermediate host: Host in which a parasite passes through the larval or asexual stages of development.

Intussusception: Telescoping of one part of an intestine into another part just distal to it.

L_3: Third-stage larva. Most often the infective stage of a parasitic helminth.

Larva: Immature stage in the life cycle of a parasite.

Metamorphosis (complex): In the development of a parasite, the form that hatches from the egg is entirely different from the adult.

Metamorphosis (simple): In the development of a parasite, the form that hatches from the egg. Resembles the adult, but is not sexually mature.

Micropyle: Opening in the egg for entrance of the spermatozoon.

Morula: Mass of cells resulting from segmentation of an egg.

Narcotize: To induce anesthesia.

Nematode: Member of the class Nematoda, which includes the true roundworms.

Paratenic host: Host that helps spread a larval stage without further larval development.

Parthenogenesis: Reproduction from a female egg that has not been fertilized by the male.

Pathognomonic: Indicative of a specific disease, especially its characteristic signs.

Pediculosis: Infestation with lice.

Prepatent period: Period between the introduction of parasites into the body and their appearance in the host's blood or tissues.

Prepatent period: Period between the introduction of parasites into the body and their appearance in the host's blood or tissues.

Primary host: Final host in which the parasite reaches sexual maturity.

Proglottid: Segment of a tapeworm containing male and female reproductive organs.

Pruritus: Severe itchiness.

Pupa: Immature stage of development of an insect.

Purgative: Agent that causes watery evacuation of the intestinal contents. Some agents produce violent evacuation of the bowels.

Rostellum: Fleshy protrusion on the cranial end of scolex of a tapeworm bearing one or more rows of spines or hooks.

Scolex: The portion of a tapeworm, the so-called head, by which it attaches itself to the wall of the host's intestine.

Scouring: Colloquial term for diarrhea in large animals.

Secondary host: Intermediate host.

Segment: Part or section of an organ or body.

Spore: Reproductive cell of lower organisms.

Sporocyst: Sac containing spores or reproductive cells.

Sporozoite: Spore formed after fertilization.

Sporozoon: A protozoan belonging to the subphylum Sporozoa.

Spurious parasite: Not a true or genuine parasite.

Transport host: Host that carries the larval stage, but in which no development occurs. This host is not necessary to complete the life cycle. Same as a paratenic host.

Trematode: A fluke; a parasitic flatworm belonging to the class Trematoda.

Vector: An animal, usually an arthropod (insect or tick), that transmits the causative organisms of a disease. In parasitology, the vector could be a paratenic host or an intermediate host.

Index